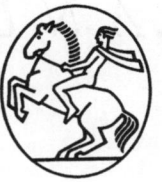

Intensivmedizinisches Seminar

K. Lenz, A. N. Laggner (Hrsg.)

Band 6

Springer-Verlag Wien New York

Patient Data Management in Intensive Care

K. Lenz, P. G. H. Metnitz (eds.)

Springer-Verlag Wien New York

Prof. Dr. Kurt Lenz, Wien
Prof. Dr. Anton N. Laggner, Wien

Prof. Dr. Kurt Lenz, Wien
Dr. phil. et Dr. med. Philipp G. H. Metnitz, Wien

© 1993 Springer-Verlag/Wien

Printed on acid-free paper

With 24 Figures

ISSN 0936-8507
ISBN-13:978-3-211-82513-6   e-ISBN-13:978-3-7091-9320-4
DOI: 10.1007/978-3-7091-9320-4

Preface

During the past decade multiform Patient Data Management Systems were planned by scientific institutions and the industry. Many of them had only a short life, some of them were developed further and are now used in clinical practice.

Motivations for the development of patient data management systems were numerous, the most pressing arose from the information overload, leading to difficulties not only for the unexperienced but also experienced intensivist facing the continuous flow of data and appropriately reacting in a time constraint, critical situation.

The aim of the First International Patient Data Management Workshop, organized during the 11th Vienna Intensive Care Days (WIT 93), was to give an overview on Patient Data Management Systems (PDMS) used in clinical practice in Europe. The most important lectures held at this workshop are published in this book. It should give information about today's facilities of PDMS and help the individual customer (intensive care physician) to decide, which system is most likely qualified to satisfy the special demands of the Intensive Care Unit he is working in.

P. G. H. Metnitz, K. Lenz   Vienna, August 1993

Contents

I. Patient Data Management Systems in Europe

Patient Data Management Systems in Europe – A Comparative Study

P. G. H. Metnitz and **K. Lenz**

Department of Inner Medicine IV, Intensive Care Unit,
University of Vienna, Austria

1. Introduction

The development of new technologies for diagnostic and therapeutic purposes in intensive care combined with the introduction of microprocessor technology has led to an enormous increase in data collection at ICUs [1, 2]. We have already reached a point where the manual handling of these amounts of data is very hard to manage [3]. The comparison of a hospital with a bank [4] by Groom and Harris in 1990 has become famous in this context. To measure the computing demands of a hospital, they looked at the number of transaction performed daily. They found that a hospital with an average census of 300 beds had the same amount of transactions as a state-wide bank with 150 branches. Further they tried to locate the demands of different units. 60% of the computing power, according to Groom and Harris, are needed by data intensive units, such as operating theatres, ICUs and laboratories (Fig. 1).

For almost a decade, computerized systems have been claimed to be the solution for handling those data. One of the reasons why the bank in our example has already computerized its transactions, but hospitals have not, is the difference in data processing budgets: The proposed 150-branch bank has a yearly budget of 52 million dollars for this purpose. No hospital can afford this. Recent technological innovations – influenced primarily by development of more sophisticated, faster and cheaper computer systems – permitted the evolution also of more

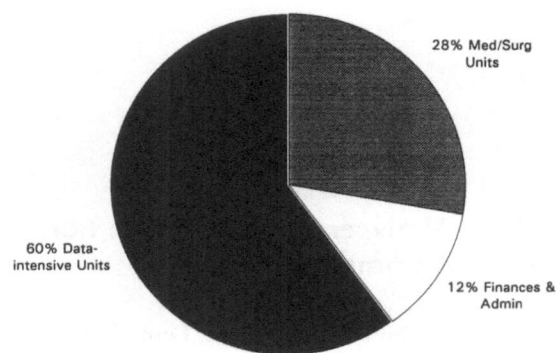

Fig. 1. Typical distribution of database transactions in a 300-patient hospital

affordable systems for Patient Data Management, so called PDM-Systems, or short PDMS.

Even though so called PDMS have been available for over a decade, their costs in combination with a lack in functionality and usefulness impeded a widespread of these systems. Since there are already some installations in Europe, there must be some arguments strong enough to explain the interest in these systems even in this developing period. Here are some of them:

- Actuality of collected data

Through connecting peripheral devices to the PDMS the measured data can be sent directly to the system, thus they are immediately available.

- Combination of various chronologically and locally
  different data

Usually, patient data are collected continually during day and night, at different times and various places: e.g. laboratories, monitors, etc. To merge and form them to a meaningful picture of the patient's condition, sophisticated paper forms have been in use until today. Yet, with the increasing amount of collected data it becomes more and more impossible to combine them in a clear way.

- New way of data presentation and review

At first, related data can be presented together, even if they come from different devices. Second, there are different ways of presenting data on a computer display: as numeric values or as charted values; Because the amount of numeric data which can be displayed on a screen in a useful way is limited, graphical displays provide the users with more information at a single glance. Moreover, reviewing data by choosing a time interval (of e.g. 12 hours or 3 days or 1 week) and evaluating the changes for this period as accurately as desired (for on-line acquired data down to one minute) gives you a very different approach. Some intensivists using such a feature report an enhanced accuracy and better personal impression, whenever the assessment of a patient's condition is necessary [5]. Third, it is also possible to arrange different interesting combinations of data sets. Blood pressure for example or oxygenic saturation could be combined with care actions to filter out artefacts. Depending on the system, the possibilities of displaying data graphically are still quite different. As development of the systems progresses, those capabilities will certainly be enhanced in future.

- Database functions

Basically a PDMS represents a database application, which implies easy accessibility of the data for scientific use. This means elimination of the time consuming work of data research in written documentation and data entry into computer programs. With a simple query it should be possible to extract the relevant data, export them into scientific calculation and plotting programs for any further analysis or interpretation desired. This would open up new horizons in carrying out studies on ICUs. In fact, up to now manufacturers have hardly taken this aspect of data processing into account. Yet there is no single installation of a PDMS in Europe which provides easy access to such use of the collected data sets. Since such a feature is essential, we hope it will soon be available. In fact we are working on that problem ourselves.

- Quality control

The use of PDMS provides a new, statistical approach to quality assurance and control: there is a lot of material – as mentioned above – for retrospective studies, e.g. for surveillance of the therapies. This could lead to an improvement in therapeutic regimes and thus be useful for the patients. Quality control concepts will also provide a basis for inter-Unit comparisons over comparable patient populations [6].

• Calculations

Of course it is possible to use the sampled data not only for display, but also for a number of useful calculations, e.g.:

—   hemodynamics: CO/CI, SV/SVI, SVR/SVRI, PVR/PVRI, LVSW/
     LVSWI, DO2/DO2I, VO2/VO2I a.o.
—   pulmonary function: Qs/Qt, AaDO2, AaDO2/FiO2, PaO2/FiO2
     a.o.
—   renal function: Creatinine clearance, FE_{Na}, a.o.
—   scores: APACHE, GCS, CHILD, TISS a.o.
—   balance: input/output, a.o.

Because these calculations have to be done for every patient they require some time and effort. In a PDMS connected to the laboratory system of the hospital, the Creatinine clearance for example could be calculated entirely automatically. This implies also that errors in calculation which occur mainly during critical periods could be avoided. Last but not least, the same data sets can be used in different calculations without the need to enter them more than once.

• Time saving

This is a slogan often used by vendors for marketing purposes. Most of the ICUs in Europe have a deficiency of nurses, so time saving mechanisms are of course a main interest of hospital management. Use of PDM-systems can in fact lead to some time saving, as users of such system report. This occurs in all situations where time consuming applications are taken over by the PDMS, like – as just stated – calculations, but also if connections to a bloodgas laboratory are available, especially on larger ICUs. Different authors report different amounts of time saved, the periods being around 30 minutes and more per day and nurse [7, 8].

• Documentation

An aspect which is primary very important in America is the presence of a proper and complete documentation:

"Complete information in a medical chart is the best defence against malpractice lawsuits. The phrase 'if it wasn't charted, it wasn't done' is famous in the lexicon of malpractice lawsuits." [9]

It is quite sure that printed documentation is very helpful in some ways, but it is also sure that with the progress of computerization this sentence will also become true in European countries: the more the possibility of recording all of the patients data will be available, the more it will be demanded by the legislators.

• Economy

Economy is matched with the already mentioned cost effectiveness. Through the use of computerized systems it has become possible to determine the costs for a patient. Typically, this is an important item in the USA too, because the private insurances keep book over the estimated therapy costs in every hospital. Hospitals with a better cost / effectiveness ratio are preferred, of course. With a PDMS the patient's data could be used to determine the costs of his stay in the ICU [10]. One of the tested PDM-systems [11] provides already a statistical database after discharging the patient, including the feature of calculating the costs of the patient's stay.

The interest in the European situation, which will increase even more in accordance to the falling prices, was the base of our study. This interest resulted from our own experience with PDMS, which led us to the following conclusions:

— At the moment PDMS are still quite expensive.
— Every system has its own specifications, advantages and disadvantages.
— A system which does not meet the local demands can not give satisfactory results when installed.
— If you buy a computer system a lot of secondary considerations are necessary: do the existing devices, e.g. ventilators, have declared interfaces? Would it be possible to connect the PDMS with the hospital's laboratory system? Therefore the decision about purchasing a PDMS should be done considerately.
— Last but not least, we found a deficiency in communication between physicians, informatic specialists and hospital managements. Normally neither physicians nor managing directors are experts in medical informatics (and why should they be), but they often decide which system is being purchased. Some companies may not be dissatisfied with this situation: it is easier for them to fascinate people who do not know much about limitations and complications of computer systems, which is in fact a very large field.

— The flow of information was quite not satisfactory: it was rather hard to separate information from advertising. A considerate decision can only be based on accurate data. Available were only those papers which are produced periodically by the public relations departments of the vendors. This kind of information may be very vivid and colourful but it always stops before touching negative aspects. To overcome this lack of information and to give an overview covering the situation of PDMS especially in Europe, was the primary goal of our work. Thus we tried to compare already installed, commercially distributed systems with regard to their specifications, functions and performance.

2. Patient Data Management Systems – Definition and Concepts

In this work we call only those systems a Patient Data Management System, in short: PDMS, which are used to supervise patients in an ICU. Especially computer systems which manage primarily administrative data are not included. This is done in contribution to the international usuance, where the term PDMS is used to characterise a system for managing patient data in ICUs. Although this provides some selection, there are still a lot of different systems which claim to be PDM-systems. Principally they can be divided into three classes:

— At first the self-made systems: especially in Germany there are a lot of very innovative groups which are working on hospital communication and computing. There exist interesting systems which provide their users with valuable information. The range starts at simple text based DOS applications and goes up to complex, GUI [12] based Windows, UNIX or even Apple applications. Though some are designed also for data management on ICUs, they are very specific to their local situation and can therefore hardly be transferred to any other location [13].
— Second, there are some minimal PDMS available: these systems are commercially available and are mostly PC based systems, which collect the information from the SDN-net (monitors) and eventually from the clinic laboratory. We call them minimal applications, because most of them don't support bedside workstations.

They are a cheap solution for small ICUs or supervising stations which do not need bigger systems for data management [14].
— Third, the commercially available bedside based PDMS which we tried to compare in this study. Yet the biggest applications and the fastest systems available today are not sufficient enough to cover the demands of managing information in an ICU. Think of further applications, such as bedside computer monitors display- ing X-rays of the patient, this and other picture based applica- tions will need even much more computer power than today's system have. Standards, like the just released MPEG [15] com- pression standard for moving pictures, will allow further develop- ment. Only systems which match international standards will be able to survive in the market.

The future of ICU computing is therefore not to be found in the first two groups. Thus we selected only bedside based systems, which had to provide following informations:

— At least one installation and commercial availability in Europe;
— Bedside based design;
— Realization on international standards, which means
  — on the hardware side on PCs or workstations,
  — on the software side e.g. on a DOS, UNIX, OS/2 Operating system;
— Minimum of functionality: the systems should be able to fulfill following functions:
  — on-line acquiring of data, e.g.: monitor data (HR, RR, SaO2, CVP),
  — managing relevant patient data, like laboratory, bloodgases,
  — display of these data on the screen,
  — report functions: printout of the patients data,
  — calculations: hemodynamics.

Following systems were available at the starting point of our study and were in compliance with those demands:

ATLANTIS – Hospitronics
CAREVUE – Hewlett Packard
CHARTMASTER – SpaceLabs

CLINICOMP – Marquette
CLINISOFT – CLINISOFT Corp.
EMTEK – Siemens

We could not get any data from the Austrian vendor of the SpaceLabs system, DRÄGER. The reason for this, according to DRÄGER, was that SpaceLabs did not want to provide any potential customer with data of the system before finishing the development. Another company selling a system potentially to be tested refused to supply us with information, Kontron.

Due to the fact that an understanding of the differences between the systems compared depends also on an insight into their technical concepts and since not every physician is an expert technician, we would like to give you a short overview over today´s PDMS concepts. Computer experienced users may forgive the simplifications done for this purpose.

Hardware

First we have to distinguish between centralized systems and decentralized systems. In a centralized system you have only one "intelligent" computer, which does all the work. The connected display stations (terminals) do not have any computer power. So there is one main computer, which shares its power with the terminals. Decentralized systems are networks, built up with Personal Computers or workstations. Every station is in fact a computer with resources of its own, like memory, storagemedia etc. This concept realizes what is called "spreaded power": Every system can be configured as powerful as needed. The only parameters which have to be shared are the data, which are commonly held on a file server.

Advantages of this concept include:

– with growing size the decentralized systems have a better performance because they do not need to share their power with any other stations;
– flexibility: every station can be configured according to its own needs: one station with a big colour display, another maybe even without or with only a small display, with a big or a small harddisk, with floppy drives or without ... This saves money because you do not need the same power for all purposes;

— price/performance ratio: the development of computer systems in the last decade has led to a surprising performance of micro computer systems: the performance of a PC with an Intel i486 CPU or with an DEC Alpha PC is comparable with that of Mainframe systems some years ago. And the next generation of microprocessors (Intel Pentium), already introduced, will be again much faster.

Interfaces

Are the connections between the computer and peripheral devices. There are some standardized interfaces, as for example the printer port or the display port on PCs or other systems. In the field of connection of medical devices there are still a lot of unsolved problems. Some declarations for interfacing medical devices exist already, but at the moment they seem to be no more than promises to the future. Three terms dominate the market [16]: HL-7, which is already implemented in different systems, but is more or less a vague concept for the

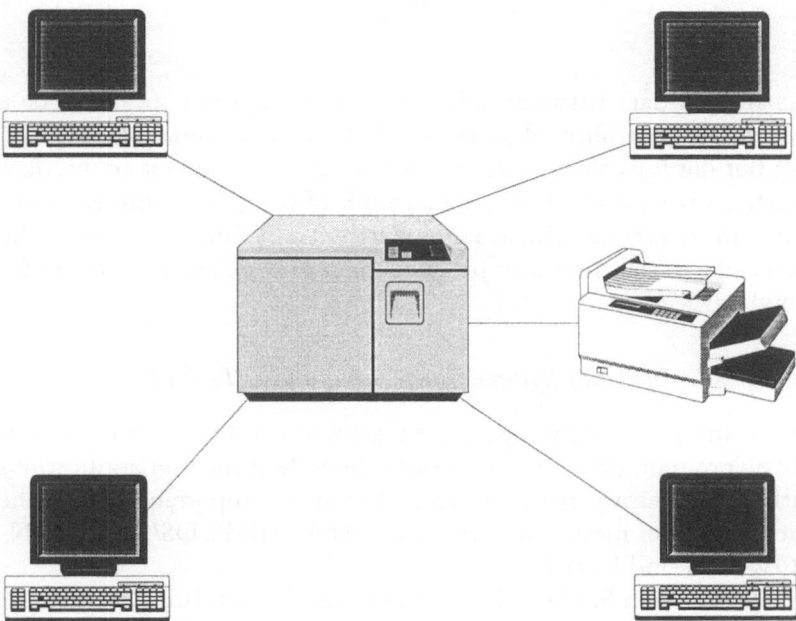

Fig. 2. Example for a Mainframe system with terminals

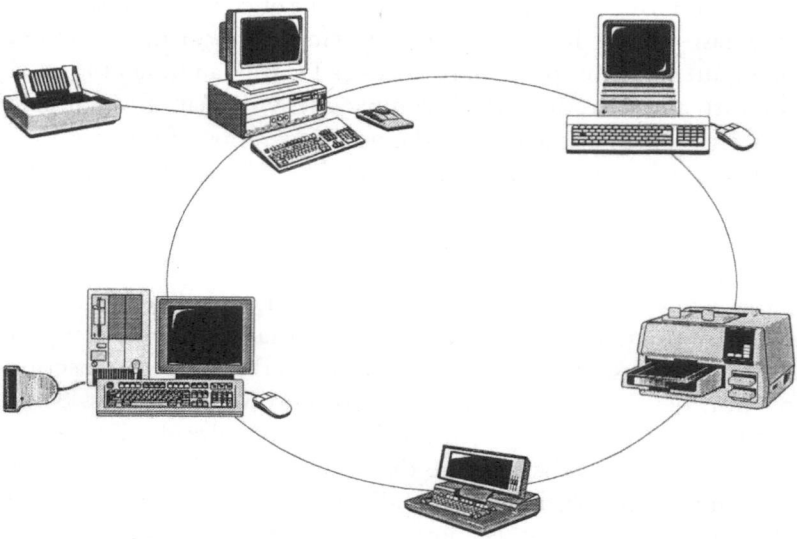

Fig. 3. Example for a decentralized computer system: workstations with different resources

exchange of data between different devices. It is not meant to be a protocol for controlling devices, which should be a domain of MEDIX. Last but not least there is also the MIB, a specification for an interface which has been worked upon for a couple of years, but is presently not in use. Insiders regard this as a problem caused by some companies, who rather like to sell their own products than provide an open system for everybody's access.

Operating Systems: Single Versus Multi Tasking

Each computer needs an operating system (short: OS) to work. This is a basic program (or a set of programs) providing the user applications with the necessary basic services. The most important OS in the microcomputer market are Microsoft's DOS, IBM's OS/2, MS WIN-DOWS NT and UNIX.

Even though MS DOS is well known as the standard OS of PCs, it is hardly a OS for PDMS. It is a single-tasking OS which means that it can handle only one task (process) at a time. In a PDMS situations may occur where multiple tasks need to be handled simultaneously, as for example data input from several devices at a time. Therefore you need a multitasking system like the other operating systems specified above. There is only one PDMS which is based on DOS as operating system, the ATLANTIS by Hospitronics. They use a so called DOS-extender (Desqview from QUEMM) to provide multitasking capability. There is also a system which uses of OS/2 from IBM: the CLINISOFT system. Though this OS has been just released in a new version, it is certainly more stable than a DOS system which provides e.g. no data security features [17].

UNIX systems have the advantage of being planned for multi-user and multi-tasking use. On the other hand they have some disadvantages, including high costs for development and administering, which requires normally the constant employment of a well trained system administrator. Another disadvantage is the existence of multiple, often incompatible versions of UNIX.

A brand-new, soon to be released operating system with exhausting features will be MS WINDOWS NT, which is already running on micro- and minicomputers from different vendors. It is compatible to DOS and WINDOWS and also some OS/2 and UNIX applications. It has already implemented network and administration features and is easy to learn and to handle. As it seems, it could be the optimal operating system for PDMS. Though the existing powerful software tools enable companies to produce complex database application in a very short time, it will be interesting to look at further developments in the PDMS market in that context.

3. The Requirements for an Optimal PDMS

The following vision of technical specifications for an optimal PDMS is to give an impression of what PDM-systems should look like. They give you a starting point for an informed comparison between those systems you might consider to purchase. Although they are not fully implemented in any of the available systems they are no pure science fiction anymore.

Hardware: Preferably a decentralized system, realized with standard PCs or workstations; they should be configured according to different requirements; user friendliness should also be provided on hardware level, which is possible e.g. through high qualitaty 16–19" displays and digital input devices such as a mouse or a bar code scanner.

Operating system: This should be hardware independent, so that different systems can be integrated according to their needs. Of course it should be a standard multi-tasking operating system with a graphical user-interface.

Network: Demands to the network depend primarily on the demands for data security and system stability. The network transmission speed should be as high as possible, otherwise problems could arise with (future-) applications which require a big amount of data to be trans-ported, such as X-ray display. Any standard LAN [18] meeting these specifications can be used.

Interfaces: All existing standards should be supported by the system, both by hard- and by software. The systems should already include drivers for the most important devices so that you can easily connect any device (plug and play) [19].

Functionality: Principally, the system should be configurable to the individual needs of the customer: free configuration of parameters, calculations, menu options, menu lists, review displays etc.

Information arrangement: On one hand, the data should be clearly arranged for easy review. On the other hand this feature should not conflict with the speed of information delivery.

Data security: All necessary actions to provide maximum level of data security should be obvious. This includes server duplexing, UPS [20], automatic data archiving and more. Password protection on different levels for read, write and system administration are a must.

Scientific use of data: An automatic copy of selected patient data should be copied on-line to a scientific SQL database, which can afterwards easily be queried by SQL front end tools, e.g. from a PC.

Connection to CIS: The data exchange between the ICU and the clinical information systems (e.g. at admission or discharge) should work without problems.

Service and support: The implementation should be performed together with the afflicted personnel. Sufficient training should be guaranteed and is the base for getting familiar with the system. A round the clock service and support contract should be signed if the hospital can not provide a service at all times.

Price/performance ratio: This should be well balanced. High prices are still an obstacle for many hospitals to buy a PDMS. Standardizations, for example in the field of data exchange or device interfacing, would of course reduce the amount of time and resources needed for development of such systems and therefore reduce the price.

4. Questionnaire for System Analyses

The goal of our study was to give an overview of the European situation in PDMS. To make the different systems comparable, we first tried to distill important criteria which determine the usefulness and practicability of such a system. Proceeding from this starting point we designed a questionnaire, which we sent to the vendors. To be part of our study, they had to answer all of our questions as profoundly as possible. The answers to our questions are gathered in the following chapter SYSTEM ANALYSIS. The reason for this was to filter out reality from advertising to get the most accurate information about the systems.

Although we designed this questionnaire to get detailed informations about the systems from the vendors, our questions are not only useful in that context. To us they seem to be equally interesting for people who will have to make decisions about purchasing a PDMS. Therefore we will not only list our questions, but also try to explain why we think they are important. If someone wants to get information about a PDMS he is normally interested in the usefulness of this system, which is represented by following criteria:

- functionality
- user friendliness
- expandability
- reliability
- data security
- support by the vendor.

They are characterized by several properties which lead towards the following questions:

I. Functionality

I.I. Included functions
— What kind of data is the system able to manage;
— possible calculations (e.g. hemodynamics, scoring) included;
— is it feasible to change the settings described above, e.g. can new parameters easily be configured by the customer or can new calculations be added (a new score system, for instance)?

I.II. Quality of data arrangement
This is an important property which has much influence on the work with the system. For instance, the speed of information delivery can be very important in critical situations. Besides, the speed of the system and therefore the amount of time needed for data entering and display is a major determinant of the system's acceptance [21].
I.II.I. Quality of the computer monitor;
I.II.II. data arrangement on screen: it is important for easy review;
I.II.III. speed of information supply.

II. User friendliness

This criterion comprises the entirety of the possibilities of interaction between the user and the system. Properties like the size of the display, graphical resolution, input devices (e.g. a mouse or trackball), the place where the system resides etc. play an immense role. User friendliness is in fact characterized though the practicability of the system during all days work. This is reflected by following facts:

II.I. Initial period
How long do the users (physicians, nurses) need to get familiar with the system? This is a very important question on ICUs, on one hand because this period falls into normal work, on the other hand because especially ICUs have an increased staff turn over.

II.II. Time saving
It is one of the most frequently proposed arguments in vendors advertising. The subjective estimation of afflicted persons, who have

already been changing to computer based documentation might provide you with certain values. If you hear about such positive results, you always should consider that there are a lot of facts which have a great impact on such an outcome:

— First, a time saving effect may need some time to establish. This is due to the fact, that the adaptation of paper based to computerized documentation can be a prolonged process;
— the type and configuration of the PDMS;
— the type and amount of peripheral devices;
— the way routine work is organized; Yet, this is quite an unexplored field. You should be aware of thinking about a PDMS as "just another device". In fact, there will be great changes in the way work is done once a PDMS is installed. The different kind of data organization provided through the use of a PDMS needs new strategies to manage. This is an area which has yet been completely ignored by the vendors. To improve the interaction between the PDMS and the users there is still a lot of clarification to be done.

III. Expandability

The performance of a PDMS depends essentially on the possibility of cooperation with peripheral devices such as monitors or ventilators. One of the main aims for a PDMS is the gathering of data from different devices, as already stated. In this context it is very important whether the vendor of the PDMS supports only devices from special companies (for example, their own), or if it is easily possible to connect to any devices. This depends on different facts:

III.I. Does the PDMS support any international standard interfaces?
E.g. RS232, MIB, HL-7, MEDIX, others.

III.II. Device drivers
The interfaces won't work alone, they need special programs which tell the computer system how to handle the transmitted data, so called "device drivers". For each device you will need a seperate driver.
III.II.I. Which drivers (this means for which devices) are included in the system?

III.II.II. Are there any other drivers available?

III.II.III. Is the vendor able to program new drivers if necessary?

III.III. Vendor dependency

Do hard- and software have to be bought together? Is it possible to buy only the software from the PDMS vendor and for example choose from different hardware manufacturers, or is it possible to use an existing hardware potential?

IV. System reliability

The reliability of a PDMS is also determining the useability. Especially in Units whose documentation is already completely computerized, systems with multiple hang-ups can cause severe problems when information is needed, but not available in critical situations. Reliability as such can be described as the efficiency of the entire security features. One criterion easily realized by the user is the count and duration of system hang-ups. As you will be able to imagine, it is hard to get any accurate data representing this problem.

V. Data reliability and data security

V.I. Fault recognition at manual data entry

The reliability of manually entered data is very important because you should be able to believe what you see on the screen. So, how are entered data checked by the system?

V.II. Data validation during on-line acquisition of data

Are the data validated automatically, or has there to be manual validation?

This inflects indeed the on screen representation of data. If the data are transferred to the PDMS automatically, e.g. every minute or every five minutes, you get a data collection which enables the system to present these data as a graphical trend. If the system needs manual validation you get a smaller amount of data, e.g. monitor data: if you validate them as usually done once or twice an hour, you get one or two points per hour on your screen. Even if you connect these points with lines they are by far not accurate enough to represent any trend. On the contrary, manual validation supplies the possibility to filter out artefacts through the need of confirmation. This is normally not done during automatic validation since no artefact recognition algorythms exist yet.

V.III. Data storage

The mechanism of data storage controls the authorized and non authorized access to the data, thereby influencing data security. Storage can be done on a local workstation, on more than one workstation (data mirroring) or on a file server (or a pair of file servers) [22].

V.III.I. Temporary storage

Locally or somewhere in the network (e.g. file server)?

V.III.II. Archiving

How long are the patient data being stored in the system? Will it later be possible to access those data sets? (that means, is it possible to look at the patient data in the same way, not only in some restricted ways?)

V.IV. Data security

Is it possible that unauthorized persons have access to patient data?

VI. Implementation and support

This includes all the services which should be provided by the vendor during and after installation. They being offered or not makes at least a big difference in the price/performance ratio. So the questions you should clarify are if and how long these services are included in the system price.

VI.I. Configuration

Is it possible to adapt the system to the individual needs of the customer during implementation?

VI.II. Changes of configuration

Is it easily possible to change the configuration after installation, or does that mean a lot of trouble? Is there any guarantee given for developing the application further and delivering program updates?

VI.III. Training

How many persons will be trained for how long? If you perceive at a later point that the training has not been sufficient, can you obtain some more?

VI.IV. Service and problem support

How fast will malfunctions be repaired? How long does the vendor supply system warranty? What are the costs of support features offered, what do they include (especially when will they be available: only on working days or also on Sundays, only during daytime or also at night, etc.).

VI.V. System maintenance

Who will be responsible for system maintenance (e.g. the hospital's computer department or the vendor or a private company)?

5. System Analyses

Data presented in this chapter were the answers which we got from the different corporations. As systems are developing (hopefully), some data may have changed during publishing this book, although we tried to update as much information as possible.

5.1. SIEMENS: EMTEK System 2000

1. Hardware
1.1. Server
SUN SPARCstation 2 with 32 MB Ram and 2 × 600 MB hard disks.

1.2. Workstations
SUN Microsystems Workstation SPARCstation IPC
24 MB Ram, 207 MB harddisk.

1.3. Displays / Resolution
SUN-19", monochrome or colour, 1192 × 900 pixel.

1.4. Network specifications
Ethernet.

2. Software
2.1. Operating system
SUN/OS (UNIX) version 4.1.2.

2.2. Applications environment
Openlook / X11

2.3. Database
SYBASE

2.4. Network specifications
TCP/IP protocol / NFS

3. Interfaces
3.1. Already implemented interfaces
HL-7 for connection onto lab devices and CIS systems.

3.2. Planned Interfaces
Eventually EDIFACT.

3.3. Device drivers
Following drivers are available at the moment:
Monitoring: Siemens, Marquette, HP, SpaceLabs, Nihon Koden.
Respiration: Siemens Servo 900 C/D, Dräger Evita, Puritan Benett.
Pumps: Imed, Ivac in preparation.
It is also possible to program drivers if the peripheral device has a declared interface (RS232).

4. Security features
System 2000 is a decentral system, which means that there is no specific server. Instead the system uses data distribution over local stations (100% redundancy). Therefore the data can be accessed even if one station fails. On the necessary administration server only network functions and interfaces, e.g. laboratory, are processed.

5. Data security and reliability
5.1. Fault recognition at manual data entry
First, data have to be validated with a password before being accepted by the system. With this password it is possible to reconstruct the person who entered the data. Second, it is possible to define minimum and maximum borders for specific data sets, which are displayed during entering data and cause an alarm if being over- or under-scored.

5.2. Data validation during on-line acquisition
Data which are sent from a peripheral device are held for 48 hours. During this time it is possible to take over the data through validation.

5.3. Data storage
5.3.1. Temporary storage
The patient data are stored locally and are mirrored on another work-

station. The capacity of the harddisk should be high enough to store a patient year.

5.3.2. Archiving
Possible with streamers since this version.

5.4. Scientific use of PDMS data
With a so called knowledge workstation, it is possible to create a scientific database which can be queried on-line (during normal systems work).

6. Data security
Password protection.

7. Configuration
Together with a team of physicians as well as nurses.

8. Support
8.1. Training
For system administrators: 3 weeks, for users: through administrators.

8.2. Service
A service contract has to be sealed.

8.3. Problem support
24 hour hotline is included in the service contract.

9. Installations
Europe: Dortmund, Städtische Kliniken, Chirurgie.
America: more than 20 installations.

5.2. MARQUETTE: CLINICOMP

1. Hardware
1.1. Server
Dual Symmetrical Multiprocessing (SMP) Unix systems with UPS. Redundant systems, synchronized on transaction basis; Intel 486, (2-6 CPUs), 16-320 MB RAM, 512 KB Cache per CPU, 64 bit bus, 28 MIPS per CPU, SCSI IF for max. 4x 316 MB, 632 MB, 1250 MB disks, optical disk, Juke box, DAT.

1.2. Workstations
No workstations, but terminals.

1.3. Displays / Resolution
19" monitor, 1280 × 1024 pixels, monochrome or colour.

1.4. Network specifications
10BaseT Unshielded Twisted Pair, 10Base2 Thin LAN. Backbone: Thick LAN, Fibre Optic and ANSI X3T9.5 compliant FDDI.

2. Software
2.1. Operating system
AT&T UNIX system V Release 3.2 (SVID) 3.

2.2. Applications environment
CCIDB (CLINICOMP Intel. Database) with CQL (Clinical Query Language) developed from LISP.

2.3. Database
See 2.2.

2.4. Network specifications
IEEE 802.E Ethernet.

3. Interfaces
3.1. Already implemented Interfaces
Clinical Data Link (CDL) HL- 7, version 2.1, CIS Link Media: RS232, RS422, Ethernet.

3.2. Planned Interfaces
MIB.

3.3. Device drivers
Following drivers are available at the moment: (see under 9.: list of installations):

Marquette, Siemens, HP, SpaceLabs, Mennen, Ventilators, IV Pumps, Urimeter, Mass Spectrometer, gas monitors. It is also possible to program specific drivers if the peripheral device has a declared interface.

4. Security features
Duplexed Servers with separate uninterruptable power supply. (40 min
to 3 hours). All devices are connected by so called "bridge repeaters".
Automatic start up of the terminals.

5. Data security
5.1. Fault recognition at manual data entry
Conditions for data entry.

5.2. Data validation during on-line acquisition
Alarm limits, software driven bidirectional protocols (like X-modem,
for example).

5.3. Data storage
5.3.1. Temporary storage
Duplexed databases.

5.3.2. Archiving
Via digital link to an external optical disk, Juke box or DAT.

5.4 Scientific use of PDMS data
On-line with form generators which sends the extracted data on to a
remote computer; (not installed in Europe at the moment).

6. Data security
Password protection on different levels: application level, workstation
level, user level; for write/read/edit/store.

7. Configuration
The configuration of the system is drafted out with the aid of a
configurations team consisting of physicians and nurses.

8. Support
8.1 Training
Local training, administrator courses and on-line help.

8.2. Service
The CLINICOMP system must be connected with the CLINICOMP
Message Centre over telephone-line or X-25; in case of malfunction the
system automatically calls this centre.

8.3. Problem Support
Service contracts with local service are possible.

9. Installations
Swedish Med.Centre., Denver:
47 displays, I/F: Siemens mon., Puriton Benett vent., ADT lab.
Univ.Hosp., Antwerp, Belgium:
52 Displays, I/F: Marquette monitors, ADT, AGB lab.
Naval Hospital, San Diego:
247 Displays, I/F: 900 Vent., HP monitors.
Sharp Memorial, San Diego:
60 Displays, I/F: HP monitors, ADT lab., Pharmacy, CIS with HL-7.
Bellevue Hospital, New York:
60 Displays, I/F: HP Mon., Puriton Benett vent., 500 Inf. pumps.
VA Medical Centre, Dallas:
26 Displays, I/F: Marquette Mon., lab., ADT with Ethernet HL-7.
Lee Mem. Hospital, Ft. Myers:
180 Displays, I/F: HP Mon., CIS, lab, Vent. Nelcor NiSaO2.
Madigan Army MedC.Tacoma:
288 Displays, I/F: Marquette Mon., Puriton Benett, vital Metrics
Urotak, IVAC pumps, Doppler Utras.IF/Out., Infrasonics Vent.

5.3. HOSPITRONICS: ATLANTIS

1. Hardware
1.1. Server
PC 386 or 486, 16 MB Ram, 210–650 MB harddisk.

1.2. Workstations
PC 386 or 486, 8 MB Ram, 120–210 MB harddisk.

1.3. Displays / Resolution
VGA.

1.4. Network specifications
Ethernet or Token Ring.

2. Software
2.1. Operating system
MS DOS 5.0.

2.2. Applications environment
QUEMM 386, Desqview.

2.3. Database
Internal format as described in the documentation.

2.4. Network specifications
Novell Netware 3.11 or higher.

3. Interfaces
3.1. Already implemented Interfaces
At the moment only communication via RS232 and RS422 is
supported.

3.2. Planned Interfaces
HL-7, MEDIX.

3.3. Device drivers

Following drivers are available at the moment:

Biomed	Bioimpedance Cardiac Output
Braun	Infusomat, Dianet/Perfusor
CDI	Blood gas analysis for Bypass
Cobe	Heart lung machine
Critikon	Dinamaps
Datex	Cardiocap, Capnomac, Multicap, Oscar, Satellite
Dräger	Anemone, Evita, Cicero, Mondine, PM8010, Narkomed 2 and 3
Engström	Elsa
Hamilton	Veolar
HP	Monitors series 78xxx
Kontron	7210
Marquette	Monitors series 701, MBX, mass spectrometer
Mennen	Horizon
Nellcor	Pulsoximeter
Ohmeda	Pulsoximeter, EtCO2
Physio-Control	Pulsoximeter
Puritan Bennet	7200 Ventilator
Siemens	Data Bus (SCM 990), 1280, 960
SpaceLabs	PCMS monitors

Spectramed	SvO2
Stockert Shiley	Heart lung machine
Vitalmetrics	Urine monitor

When – for a special installation – drivers are required which have to be programmed, they are included in the systems price – if the devices are known at the time of the offer. If a client needs new drivers for an existing version he has to provide the interface protocol; in this case the costs are individually calculated. A device driver development kit is also available.

4. Security features
UPS, Backup [23], or other security mechanisms have to be done by the user.

5. Data security
5.1. Fault recognition at manual data entry
Manually entered data are checked whether they deviate from a defined minimum or maximum level.

5.2. Data validation during on-line acquisition
No answer.

5.3. Data storage
5.3.1. Temporary storage
Patient data are locally stored every two minutes and can be moved to the server in any user definable interval.

5.3.2. Archiving
After discharging the patient, the data set is stored on the server in ASCII format. Any other organization of archiving has to be done by the user.

5.4. Scientific use of PDMS data
The ASCII data can be converted into any of the existing database applications.

6. Data security
Has to be administered by the user.

7. Configuration
The configuration of the system is done through the use of special configuration files, which are interpreted by the main program at start up. The client specific configuration can be done by a trained member of the user or by the vendor.

8. Support
8.1. Training / 8.2. Service
No answer.

8.3. Problem Support
Individually for every project.

9. Installations
University of Vienna, Clinic of Anaesthesiology, Department for Heart and Thorax-surgery.

5.4. HEWLETT PACKARD: CAREVUE 9000

1. Hardware
1.1. Server
HP Apollo Model 730; 66 MHz PA RISC CPU, 32 MB Ram, 2 × 440 MB SCSI hard disks and EISA slot; external 1350 MB SCSI harddisk.

1.2. Workstations
HP Apollo Model 710; 50 MHz PA RISC CPU, 16 MB Ram: diskless stations.

1.3. Display / Resolution
19" colour display with 1280 × 1024 pixel or
19" monochrome display with 1280 × 1024 pixel or
16" colour display with 1024 × 768 pixel.

1.4. Network specifications
Vendor installed LAN AUI configuration; External transceiver (MAU); Ethernet compatible.

2. Software
2.1. Operating system
HP-UX 8.07.

2.2. Applications environment
X-Windows [24], OSF/Motif.

2.3. Database
Allbase (object oriented queries on base of SQL).

2.4. Network specifications
Ethernet, Star LAN topology.
Protocol: TCP/IP.

3. Interfaces
3.1. Already implemented interfaces
Monitor data from the SDN-net over Careport station;
HL-7 is used as external data format; for exchanging data a gateway computer is needed.

3.2. Planned Interfaces
MEDIX.

3.3. Device drivers
Drivers for all HP peripherals and compatible are included in the system.

Following peripherals from different vendors are already connected to the CAREVUE:

In Austria:

Monitors:	HP CMS patient monitor (Merlin)
MT [25] devices:	Beckmann laboratory, Dräger Evita respirator, Cicero B, Ciba Corning 200 laboratory

World wide:

Monitors:	SpaceLabs, Clovers, Minishots
Respirators:	Dräger, Siemens, Puritan Bennett
MT devices:	Ohmeda, Nellcor, Bard Urimeter
Laboratories:	16 different laboratory systems. e.g.: Meditech, Burroghs, CHC, Sunquest, Cerner, SM Path Lab, DHCP;
HCIS/CIS systems:	16 different. e.g.: Proprietary systems, Gerber Alley, TDS, DHCP, Meditech, Baxter, SMS.

RS232 drivers for the gateway can be done.

4. Security features

Dual server configuration with mirrored software and database (shadowing); this guarantees data access also in the case of malfunction of one of the server systems. Uninterruptable power supplies (UPS) for both servers.

5. Data security

5.1. Fault recognition at manual data entry

Patient data are only stored after validation with user specific password.

5.2. Data validation during on-line acquisition

On-line data have to be validated manually. Starting with version F it will also be the possible to choose between manual and automatic validation. On-line data coming from MT devices can be validated manually or automatically. On-line data from laboratory information systems have to be validated there.

5.3. Data storage

5.3.1. Temporary storage

The workstations are diskless stations, data are only stored on the file servers.

5.3.2. Archiving

Archiving of patient data is not possible at the moment. It will be supported starting with version G; (current version: E).

5.4. Scientific use of PDMS data

It is possible to extract data from the system with the use of a DOS based program, called DBExport. This provides files in ASCII format, which have to be converted into a database. (Problems occur because it is only possible to query the database 72 hours backwards. For every new version of the system software you have to purchase a new DBExport, to create new queries and to adapt your existing database and converting routines!)

6. Data security

Read/Write level passwords.

7. Configuration

The configuration of the system is done by a team of physicians and nurses, conducted by a member of HP. The phase of implementation leads towards a testrun. After necessary corrections, the system is ready to start routine working.

8. Support
8.1. Training
Nurses: 2 days training for 5 nurses, who train their colleagues in turn; Physicians: 2 hours training.
System operators: half a day training for a specified system operator which is responsible for simple services on printers and workstations.
System managers: 2 days training for two people of the hospital's computer department.

8.2. Service
Hardware: 1 year starting from delivery; Software: 1 year; Later a service contract for hard- and software service should be sealed.

8.3. Problem support:
Depends on the service contract.

9. Installations
America:
22 hospitals with 397 workstations.

Europe:

Austria:	Vienna	AKH / Universitätskliniken
	Vienna	SMZ Ost
Sweden:	Stockholm	Sudersjukhuset
	Lund	University Clinics
Swiss:	Basel	Kantonspital
	Genf	HCUG Geneva
France:	Paris	Piti – Paris
	Limoges	CRU des Limoges
Great Britain:	London	Royal Brompton Hospital
	Oxford	University Clinics
	Edinborough	University Clinics
Germany:	Berlin	Universitätsklinikum Steglitz
	Leipzig	Universitätsklinikum

	Kiel	Universitätsklinikum
	Tübingen	Universitätsklinikum
	Freiburg	Universitätsklinikum
	Bochum	Bergmannsheil Klinikum
	Frankfurt	Herzchirurgisches Zentrum
Dänemark:	Oskilde	University Clinics

5.5. CLINISOFT: CLINISOFT Information System

1. Hardware
1.1. Server
IBM compatible PC-486, 32 MB Ram, 800 MB hard disks
Network adapter, Streamer.

1.2. Workstations
IBM compatible PC-486, 16 MB Ram, 120 MB hard disks
Network adapters, adapter for connection of peripheral devices.

1.3. Displays / Resolution
Any OS/2 compliant graphics adapters; e.g. 1024×768 with XGA-2
or 8514 compatible.

1.4. Network specifications
Any OS/2 compatible LAN.

2. Software
2.1. Operating system
OS/2 version 1.3; now upgrading to OS/2 V. 2.1.

2.2. Applications environment
CLINISOFT Software, MS SQL Server, MS Excel.

2.3. Database
MS SQL Server.

2.4. Network specifications
Any OS/2 compatible LAN software, e.g. MS LAN Manager, IBM
LAN server.

3. Interfaces
3.1. Already implemented interfaces
HL-7 for connection to laboratory systems.

3.2. Planned Interfaces
HL-7 for connection to different CIS.

3.3. Device drivers
Following drivers are available at the moment:
Monitoring: Siemens Sirecust, Marquette, HP, SpaceLabs, Kone 565, Datex AS/3
Ventilation: Siemens Servo 900 C/D
Infusions pumps: Braun, Ivac
Pulsoximeters: Datex Satellite, Oskar
Metabolic monitors: Datex Deltatrac
For devices with a declared interface, programming of drivers is possible.

4. Security features
On the hardware side: UPS, Disk duplexing or mirroring.
On the software side: fault tolerant net software: e.g. Novell SFT level II or higher: all transactions done in the database are recorded; after a system hang-up with errors caused in the database these recordings can be used to recover the database; this minimizes loss of data.

5. Data security
5.1. Fault recognition at manual data entry
It is possible to define "biological limits" for all parameters; the entered values are checked if they match those values.

5.2. Data validation during on line acquisition
All on line acquired data are filtered in two or five minute intervals. These medians are displayed on the PDM-monitor.

5.3. Data storage
5.3.1. Temporary storage
The storage of data is done centrally on the file servers database.

5.3.2. Archiving
Can be done with streamers or any other from the Operating system supported devices.

5.4. Scientific use of PDMS data

The data are stored in a SQL Server database; after discharging the patient a statistic database is created automatically, which provides important information about demographic values: length of stay, costs of therapy, ...

In the future it will also be possible to copy the patient data to a second scientific SQL database which can be queried with any SQL front end.

6. Data security

Password protection.

7. Configuration

One of the advantages of the system is the possibility to adapt it to the user's needs. The configuration has to be done mainly by the user. CLINISOFT supports the user by planning and supervising the installation.

8. Support

8.1. Training

The system can be delivered in any language; the first user training is done during the installation phase; Training for administrators: 3 weeks; User training: "train the trainer".

8.2. Service

A service contract has to be made; price: 15% of the software price per year including one software update per year and the membership in the users group.

8.3. Problem Support

Depends on the service contract.

9. Installations

Finland: Kuopio University Hospital
Sweden: Uddevalia Sjukhus

6. Table of Functions

Explanation

yes	this function was included in the tested system;
no	this function was not included in the tested system;
*	it is possible to configure this function, but it was not done for the tested system;
x	a special display is not available for that item; therefore the single parameters can not be shown as yes or no for that display;
Display configurable	this option means that the display can be configured by the user; e.g., new parameters can be added, unnecessary ones deleted;
CAREVUE – version E and F	during releasing this book, version E is ready to be replaced by version F; therefore the new functions provided with it are included, marked by an "F:"

SYSTEM	EMTEK vers. 3.A	CLINICOMP	ATLANTIS	CAREVUE vers. E, F	CLINISOFT
ADMISSION DISPLAY	yes	yes	yes	yes	yes
Patient data	yes	yes	yes	yes	yes
Diagnosis at admission	yes	yes	yes	yes	yes
Diagnosis	yes	yes	yes	yes	yes
Allergies	yes	yes	yes	yes	yes
Blood group	yes	yes	yes	yes	yes
Transferred from	yes	yes	no	yes	yes
Display configurable	yes	yes	no	yes	yes
GRAPHICAL PATIENT CHART	yes	yes	yes [26]	yes	no such display [27]
HR	yes	yes	yes	yes	XX
MAP	yes	yes	yes	yes	XX
SaO2	yes	yes	yes	*	XX
ETCO2	yes	yes	yes	*	XX

SYSTEM	EMTEK vers. 3.A	CLINICOMP	ATLANTIS	CAREVUE vers. E, F	CLINISOFT
Temperature	yes	yes	yes	yes	XX
Display configurable	yes	yes	yes	no	XX
VITAL PARA-METER / QUICK LOOK SCREEN	yes	yes	yes	yes	configurable
HR	yes	yes	yes	yes	*
RR	yes	yes	yes	yes	*
ABP	yes	yes	yes	yes	*
MAP	yes	yes	yes	yes	*
CVP	yes	yes	yes	yes	*
pO2	yes	yes	yes	yes	*
pCO2	yes	yes	yes	yes	*
pH	yes	yes	yes	yes	*
FiO2	yes	yes	yes	yes	*
I:E-ratio	yes	yes	yes	yes	*
Urine	no	yes	yes	yes	*
Balance	no	yes	no	yes	*
Events	yes	yes	no	*	*
Type of ventilation	yes	yes	no	yes	*
Display configurable	yes	yes	no	yes	*
RESPIRATORY SCREEN	yes	yes	yes	yes	yes
Device	yes	yes	yes	yes	yes
Type of ventilation	yes	yes	yes	yes	yes
Set values	yes	yes	yes	yes	yes
Measured values	yes	yes	yes	* [28]	yes
MBG	yes	yes	yes	yes	yes
ABG	yes	yes	yes	yes	yes
Display configurable	yes	yes	yes	yes	yes

SYSTEM	EMTEK vers. 3.A	CLINICOMP	ATLANTIS	CAREVUE vers. E, F	CLINISOFT
LABORATORY VALUES DISPLAY	yes	yes	yes	yes	yes
Electrolytes	yes	yes	yes	yes	yes
Blood chemistry	yes	yes	yes	yes	yes
Blood analysis	yes	yes	yes	yes	yes
Coagulation	yes	yes	yes	yes	yes
Bloodgas analysis	yes	yes	yes	yes	yes
Urine analysis	yes	yes	yes	yes	yes
Osmolality	yes	yes	yes	yes	yes
Immunology	yes	yes	yes	yes	yes
Micro biological tests	yes	*	no	*	*
Micro biological table of resistance	yes	no	no	no	no
Drug levels	yes	yes	yes	yes	yes
Display configurable	no	yes	no	yes	yes
MEDICATIONS SCREEN	no sep. display curr.	yes	no separate display [29]	yes	yes
Calculation of dose [30]	yes	yes	no	yes	yes
Calculation of rate [31]	yes	yes	no	yes	yes
Standard doses given	no	yes	no	yes	yes
Maximum dose alarms	yes	yes	no	yes	24-h max.
Display configurable	XX	yes	no	yes	no
BALANCE SCREEN	yes	yes	yes	yes	yes
Blood	yes	yes	yes	yes	yes
Crystalloid solutions	yes	yes	yes	yes	yes
Perfusors	yes	yes	yes	yes	yes
Infusions	yes	yes	yes	yes	yes
Enteral nutrition	yes	yes	yes	yes	yes
Parenteral nutrition	yes	yes	yes	yes	yes
Urine	yes	yes	yes	yes	yes

SYSTEM	EMTEK vers. 3.A	CLINICOMP	ATLANTIS	CAREVUE vers. E, F	CLINISOFT
Input/Output	yes	yes	yes	yes	yes
Netto balance	yes	yes	yes	yes	yes
Graphical Display of Balance	yes	at trend analyses	yes	at trend analyses	yes
Display configurable	yes	yes	no	yes	yes
TREND ANALYSES - GRAPHICAL	all param. available	all param. available	all param. available	all param. available	all param. available
HR	yes	yes	yes	yes	yes
ABP	yes	yes	yes	yes	yes
SaO2	yes	yes	yes	yes	yes
RR	yes	yes	yes	yes	yes
ETCO2	yes	yes	yes	yes	yes
Temperature	yes	yes	yes	yes	yes
Hemodynamics	yes	yes	yes	*	yes
Renal function	*	yes	yes	*	yes
Laboratory values	*	yes	yes	*	yes
Balance	yes	yes	yes	*	yes
Scores	yes	yes	yes	*	yes
Which time interval to display at once	any	any	any	maximum 48 hours	any
Display configurable	yes	yes	yes	yes	yes
DIALYSIS / EXTRACORPORAL THERAPY	*	*	*	yes	*
Modality	*	*	*	yes	*
Membrane	*	*	*	yes	*
Flow	*	*	*	yes	*
AP/VP	*	*	*	yes	*
TMP	*	*	*	yes	*
UFR	*	*	*	yes	*
Time of therapy	*	*	*	yes	*
RR-MAP	*	*	*	yes	*

SYSTEM	EMTEK vers. 3.A	CLINICOMP	ATLANTIS	CAREVUE vers. E, F	CLINISOFT
HR	*	*	*	yes	*
Dialysate K/Na	*	*	*	yes	*
Display configurable	*	*	*	yes	*
HEMODYNAMICS	yes	yes	yes	yes	yes
ABP	yes	yes	yes	yes	yes
CVP	yes	yes	yes	yes	yes
LVEF/RVEF	yes	yes	yes	yes	yes
CO/CI	yes	yes	yes	yes	yes
SV/SVI	yes	yes	*	yes	yes
SVR/SVRI	yes	yes	*	yes	yes
PVR/PVRI	yes	yes	*	yes	yes
LVSW/LVSWI	yes	yes	*	yes	yes
DO2/DO2I	yes	yes	*	yes	yes
VO2/VO2I	yes	yes	*	yes	yes
PAP	yes	yes	yes	yes	yes
PAWP	yes	yes	yes	yes	yes
Display configurable	yes	yes	yes	yes	yes
PULMONARY FUNCTION	*	yes	*	yes	yes
Qs/Qt	*	yes	*	yes	yes
AaDO2	*	yes	*	yes	yes
AaDO2/FiO2	*	yes	*	yes	yes
PaO2/FiO2	*	yes	*	yes	yes
Display configurable	yes	yes	yes	yes	yes
RENAL FUNCTION	*	*	*	yes	yes
Creatinine clearance	*	*	*	yes	yes
Free water clearance	*	*	*	yes	yes

SYSTEM	EMTEK vers. 3.A	CLINICOMP	ATLANTIS	CAREVUE vers. E, F	CLINISOFT
Fract. extraction of Na, K	*	*	*	yes	yes
Electrolyte excretion/d	*	*	no	yes	yes
UN production/day	*	*	*	yes	yes
Display configurable	yes	yes	yes	yes	yes
SCORES	yes	yes	see I.N.C.A.	yes	yes
APACHE II	*	yes	no	yes	yes
APACHE III	*	*	no	yes	*
CHILD	*	*	no	yes	*
GCS	*	yes	no	yes	yes
TISS	*	*	no	*	yes
CARE ACTIVITIES DISPLAY	yes	*	see I.N.C.A.	yes	yes
Prescriptions	no	*	no	no	yes
Medical diagnoses	yes	yes	at admission display	yes	yes
Care diagnoses	yes	yes	no	no	yes
Automatic configuration [32]	*	*	no	no	yes
Tick off already done activities	yes	no	no	no	yes
Alarm when not handled	no	no	no	no	yes
Graphical display of the body [33]	no	no	no	no	yes
Notes possible	yes	yes	yes	yes	yes
Display configurable	*	yes	no	yes	yes
NUTRITION	*	yes	no	no	no
Fluid account	*	yes	no	no	yes
Accounting of calories	no	yes	no	no	yes
Acc. of electrolytes	yes	no	no	no	yes

SYSTEM	EMTEK vers. 3.A	CLINICOMP	ATLANTIS	CAREVUE vers. E, F	CLINISOFT
DOCUMENTA-TION	*	*	no	F: yes	yes
Anamnesis report function	yes	*	no	F: yes	*
Transfer report function	yes	*	no	no	yes
Automatic take over of patient data [34]	yes	*	no	no	no
Diagnoses database	yes	*	no	no	yes
NOTES	yes	yes	yes	yes	yes
Notes per worksheet cell	yes	no	no	yes	yes
Overview for notes	yes	yes	no	F: yes	yes
Sorting notes for different criteria	yes	yes	no	no	yes
PRINTED REPORTS	all trends configur-able as reports	any report configur-able	only with module Hospiprint [35]	yes	any report configur-able
Patient chart	yes	yes	XX	yes	yes
Laboratory	yes	yes	XX	*	yes
Hemodynamics	yes	yes	XX	yes	yes
Ventilation	yes	yes	XX	yes	yes
Renal function	*	*	XX	yes	yes
Medications	yes	yes	XX	yes	yes
Pulmonary functions	*	yes	XX	yes	yes
Balance	yes	yes	XX	yes	yes
Care report	yes	*	XX	yes	yes
Complete patient file	yes	yes	XX	yes	yes
Admission data	yes	yes	XX	yes	yes
Vital parameters - quick look	yes	yes	XX	yes	yes
Extracorporal therapy	*	*	XX	yes	*

SYSTEM	EMTEK vers. 3.A	CLINICOMP	ATLANTIS	CAREVUE vers. E, F	CLINISOFT
Trend analyses	yes	yes	XX	yes	yes
Interval changeable?	yes	24 hours maximum	XX	yes	yes
DATA ACQUISITION	yes	yes	yes	yes	yes
Ward sided laboratories	yes	yes	yes	*	yes
Laboratory information systems	yes	yes	yes	*	yes
X-ray systems	from SIEMENS	no	yes [36]	*	no
ON-LINE DATA ACQUISITION	yes	yes	yes	yes	yes
Monitors	yes	yes	yes	yes	yes
Ventilators	yes	yes	yes	*	yes
Pulsoximeters	from monitor	yes	yes	*	yes
Perfusors	yes	yes	yes	*	yes
Dialysis/filtration devices	*	*	*	*	*
IABP	*	yes	*	*	*
Mechanism of data import into PDMS	validation	validation	validation	validation	validation
Manual validation	yes	yes	no	yes	no
Automatic validation	yes	no	yes	F: yes	yes
Artefact recognition	yes	no	no	no	median-filtering
Automatic validation all ... min	1 min	no	10–60 min.	F: 5–120 min.	2 or 5 min.
Storage without validation	48 h storage	no	no	no [37]	patient stay
Data acquisition from CIS	*	yes	*	*	*
Data transfer to CIS	*	yes	*	*	*

SYSTEM	EMTEK vers. 3.A	CLINICOMP	ATLANTIS	CAREVUE vers. E, F	CLINISOFT
DATA STORAGE	yes	yes	yes, in ASCII-format	currently not permanent!!	yes
In the Worksheet	no limitation	minimum 25 years	no	around 12 weeks [38]	patient stay
Archiving possible?	automatic	automatic	yes, from the user	available with ver. G	yes
DATABASE					
Scientific use of the data possible?	not installed in Europe	not installed in Europe	yes [39]	yes	in preparation
Query language	SQL	SQL-like	no	SQL-like	SQL
Database	SYBASE	CCIDB	no	ALLBASE	MS SQL Server
Scientific Database	INFORMIX, ORACLE	CCIDB	no	no	not yet
DISPLAY					
Associative displays [40]	no	no	at the balance display	no	yes
Interval configurable	yes	no	yes	yes	yes
minimal configurable interval of sections	1 min	XX	1 min	1 min	1 min
maximal configurable interval	patient stay	patient stay	patient stay	8 hours	patient stay
Configuration: done by vendor or user?	both possible	at the moment only from Marquette	user	both possible	user

7. Information Retrieval Tests

During the investigations for this study we recognized big differences in the speed of information delivery, which has a huge impact on effectivity. To evaluate the variations in performance we designed some "information retrieval tests". These were based on the assumption that a sequence of interrogations could point out those differences. In fact, we tried to choose some questions covering most parts of the tested PDMS. They are listed below and have been taken from routine work – they are questions which have been asked at shifts.

Obviously the "results" do not give accurate values, instead they could be regarded as an additional evaluation instrument which should be interpreted in the right context such as equipment, number of beds, etc. This is due to the following facts:

– First, there are big differences in the system designs. One system for example may be based mainly on numeric displays, other systems more on graphically oriented displays. The HOSPITRONICS system, e.g., consists of different modules which you can buy seperately. The ICU where we performed our tests was only fitted with the basic module ATLANTIS, which enables you to gather and manage on-line data. To handle care activities the module I.N.C.A. [41] has to be purveyed.
– Second, we had no possibility to design a "test patient" and enter his data into the different systems. This would have resulted in more exact values, of course.

---

1   Date of insertion of the central venous catheter;
2   Fluid balance of the last 5 days;
3   Sedation: dose per hour, since what time and which dose did you apply before?
4   Changes of the creatinine clearance and the free water clearance of the last 3 days;
5   Blood pressure and cardiocirculatory therapy 8 hours ago: MAP, HR, CVP, medication;
6   Adjustments of the mechanical ventilator and bloodgas analysis of the last 4 hours: FiO_2, type of ventilation, I:E, Pmax, expiratoral tidal volume, PO_2, PCO_2, pH
7   How often did the patient have a temperature over 38°C in the last 4 days?
8   Extracorporal therapy: adjustments of the last 24 hours: Flow, TMP, Heparine;
9   How often did you take bronchial specimens for culture in the last 3 days?
10 How often did the patient produce stool in the last 4 days?

Our aim was not to produce scientifically valuable results, but to give potential customers some ideas of how much the systems can differ. There are some reasons why we think that those tests are quite interesting. As we saw, there seem to be two main criteria for the outcome of those experiments:

At first the hardware used: in a PC based system, e.g., it makes a big difference if you use 386 SX-20 machines or 486 DX-66; the same happens when you use a workstation (see later the difference between Apollo 400 and 700 series); The second impact results from the system design and data arrangement: how are the data arranged? Is it easily possible to figure out important values, e.g. does the system have a seperate screen for displaying the daily balance data? The possibility to configure review screens e.g. makes it much easier to find the data needed, than to find them among a big amount of numbers.

One might think that the data of the different "tested" patients make a difference. But as we performed our tests with various patients, we realized that the patient data did not affect the outcome as much as we thought: most of the time consumed was used for changing to the appropriate display and the right time, especially in slower systems.

All tests were conducted by the same person. On the other hand we tried to locate one person which was most familiar with the system in every Unit. Every question was explained in detail before execution. Starting from a "standard screen", we measured the time required to extract the information. To make the executing people familiar with this kind of questions we created a preliminary set first. Soon after that we did the final tests. We documented the time of the beginning as well as the end of the information delivery. With that regime we got two values:

- The first one describes the time that the probationer needs to get to the right display; this gives you an overview how fast important data can be accessed. It mainly depends on the quality of data arrangement and on the configuration of the displays. Systems with one or more good review screens should have better results in this respect.
- The second value determines the time the probationer needed to extract the entire information. This characterizes mainly two parameters: the speed of the system and the kind of data display: systems with graphical data presentation had great advantages in

answering those questions which required to scroll back in time, for example questions number two, five and seven.

The results shown as graphic charts should be interpreted carefully in combination with the table of functions and the system analyses. They should not be seen as an exact statistical comparative approach but as a good tool to check the behaviour of those PDMS.

Since this year Hewlett Packard install their system on a faster hardware platform, the Apollo Series 700. We took this chance to demonstrate the enhancement of the response time. Although the new systems uses RISC CPU's, it is still one of the slowest systems tested. Hewlett Packard told us that they are working very hard on this problem, it should be solved with the next releases.

Those data series in the charts which are not filled with a bar were questions which could not be answered by the participants. This was caused by the differences between the examinated Units: we had surgical as well as medical Units in our trial; The CLINICOMP and the ATLANTIS systems did not have the care managing parts installed yet, which should also be noticed.

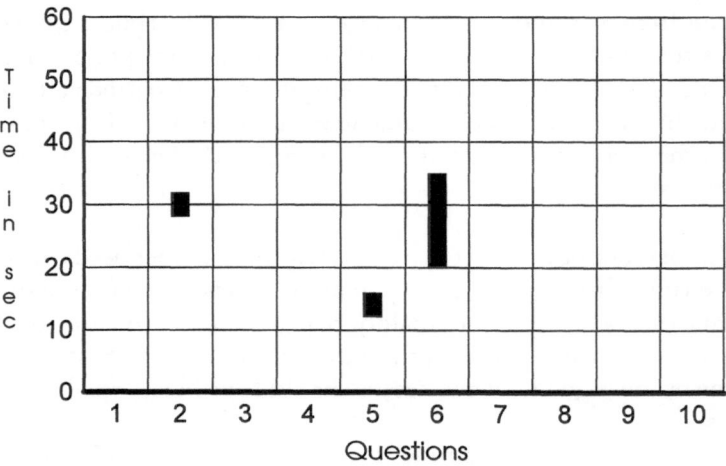

Fig. 4. Configuration: PC Network, Novell 3.11 with 22 bedside stations; Token ring. Server: PC-386 DX – 33 MHz, 8 MB RAM, 320 MB HD, OS: Novell. Workstations: PC-386 SX – 20 MHz, 8 MB RAM, 120 MB HD, OS: MS DOS 5.0

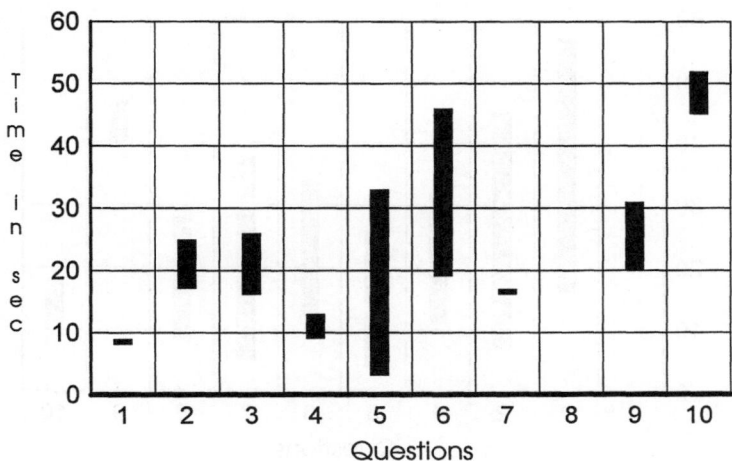

Fig. 5. Configuration: PC network, 16 bedside stations, Token ring. Server: PC 486 DX – 33 MHz, 16 MB RAM, 600 MB HD, OS: OS/2 1.3. Workstations: PC-486 SX – 25 MHz, 8 MB RAM, OS: OS/2 1.3

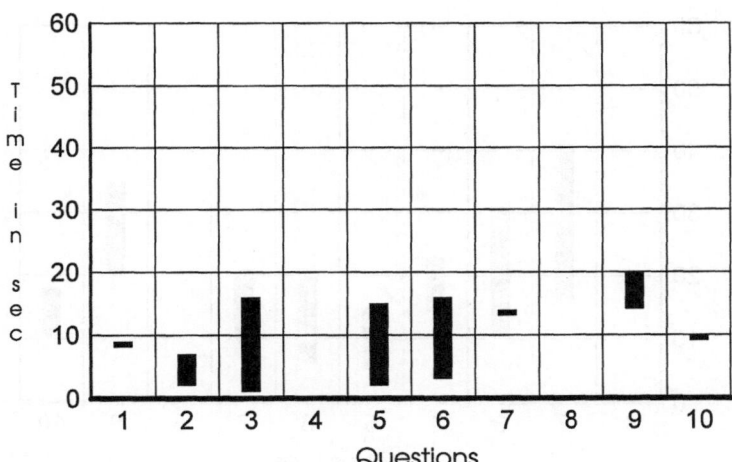

Fig. 6. Configuration: Ethernet LAN; Ring Topology; 16 bedside stations. Server: SUN SPARCstation 2 Administration server. Workstations: SUN SPARCstation IPC

P. Metnitz and K. Lenz

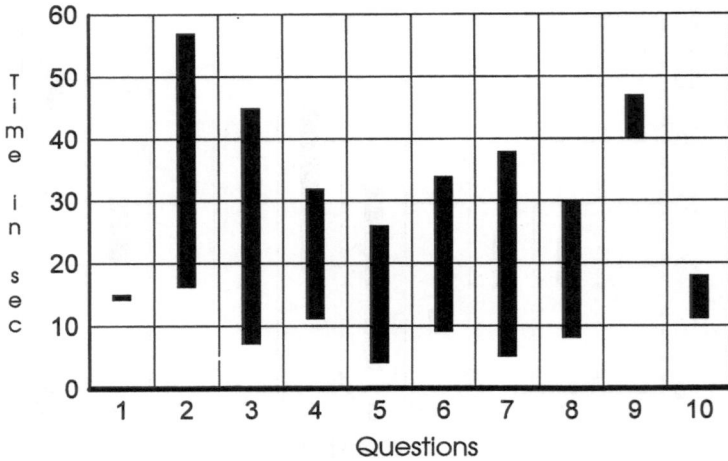

Fig. 7. Configuration: HP network; Ethernet Star LAN; 9 bedside stations. Servers: 2 HP APOLLO 400 Servers, 32 MB RAM, 1,2 GB HD, OS: HP-UX. Workstations: diskless APOLLO 400, 68030 CPU, 50 MHz, 16 MB RAM, OS: HP-UX

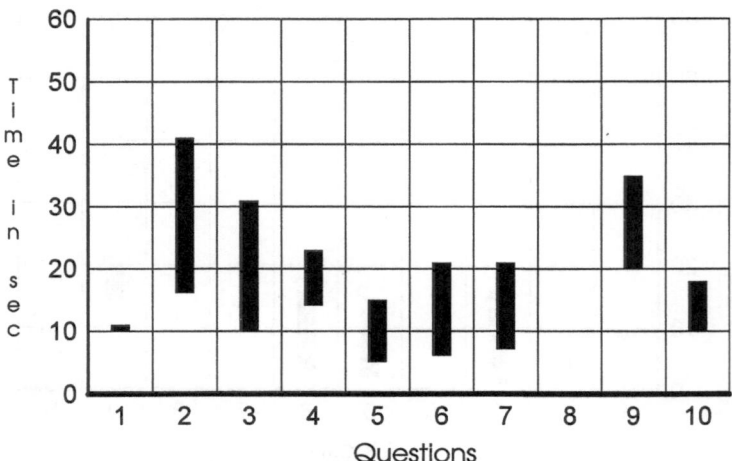

Fig. 8. Configuration: HP-network; Ethernet Star LAN; 8 bedside stations. Server: 2 HP APOLLO 700, PA RISC CPU 66 MHz, 32 MB RAM, 2,4 GB HD, OS: HP-UX. Workstations: diskless APOLLO 700, PA RISC CPU, 50 MHz, 16 MB RAM, OS: HP-UX

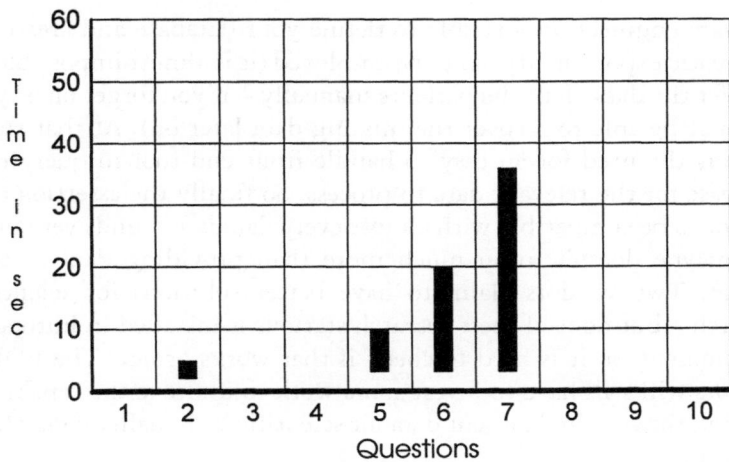

Fig. 9. Configuration: 2 Mainframes SEQUENT SYMMETRY 2000; w. 4 × i486 CPUs, 128 MB RAM, OS: UNIX. 52 Terminals connected via Ethernet

8. Conclusions

Anybody considering to buy a PDMS should know what he wants and what he needs – and what he gets. At least we would like to present some conclusions drawn from our experiences and tests.

• The preceeding pages show the variations in information delivery. As the values speak for themselves it is not necessary to give a lot of comments. But the more the work with the PDMS consumes time, the less it is used by the personnel.

• There are a lot of promises waiting to be fulfilled. For example, every vendor of a PDMS promises easy data access for scientific research – but three of the systems just have the ability to produce or export data in the well known ASCII format [42]. Those data have to be reconverted into a database format. Thus a new database has to be created (instead of using the one which already comes with the system); this is not as easy as it may seem: exporting all the data delivers a large amount of them which can only be handled with a professional database (e.g. ORACLE or MS SQL Server); for that purpose either the connection to a hospital Mainframe is needed or a workstation with quite big capacities has to be bought. Further, a software engineer who is able to define your database and create an automatic export utility has to be employed (it is almost impossible to transfer the data of all the patients manually – if you forget once, you may not be able to recover the missing data later on). At that stage there is the need for an easy to handle front end tool to query this database for the relevant data to process. So finally the assertion of a vendor to be compatible with almost every database sounds very nice, but maybe doesn't mean much more than providing data in text format. Two vendors claim to have better solutions for scientific research – but none of these research stations is installed in Europe at the moment, so it is hard to check if that works or not. The PDMS vendors will still have to invest some work to improve the capability of using the acquired patient data for scientific and quality controling purposes.

• Our analysis shows that a PDMS can only operate efficiently if it is connected to peripheral devices. PDMS which are not interfaced to any devices do not make much sense. In fact, parallel charting is actually frustrating the efforts of nurses. But the development of an interface capable to perform all necessary tasks is still a challenge. For example, there is no interface type available which is capable of controlling peripheral devices. This limitation becomes already important at a very basic level: there is no chance for a PDMS to control the transmitted data; e.g. to check if and at what time the solution infused was changed or not. At the moment it is just possible to record the amount of fluid flowing through. If a physician or a nurse is inadvertant only once during entering data you get wrong recordings. And that might impede your therapy.

• Computer systems save time. This might be true in some situations and under some conditions. Everybody who has worked with computer systems knows that this need not be true at all. Computers may save your time in some cases, but they produce work as well. Anybody who ever tried to enter a quick note into a computerized notebook, will know what we mean. Most of the times it is much quicker to do that by hand on a simple piece of paper. This might also apply to some of the care documentations, depending on the system [43]. Some nurses report an increased amount of time used for documentation. Partly, it might be due to different focuses in the system designs. Some PDMS are primarily designed for collecting on-line data, other systems have their focus especially on care documentation.

Regarding this, some centers do not attach great importance on doing the whole care documentation via PDMS.

• We found that systems with graphical data presentation have advantages over systems, which present the data only in a numeric format. A big screen filled with numbers is more an obstacle for easy reviewing than a good alternative for a paper chart. Though all of the tested systems had graphical user interfaces they were not perfect at all. Practicability and user friendliness is an item further to be enhanced. The CLINISOFT system is the first one which is primarily based on graphic displays. This provides a new and different approach to patient data. Only clinical use in routine work will proof its useability.

• This does not mean that the available PDMS are useless. But as long as the industrial partners do not produce and sell open systems which can easily communicate with devices from other vendors, as long as there are no standards defined – or even rejected by the industry, the customers have to rely upon the good will of the vendor to reduce such deficiencies. But this has to be seen as a double sided process: as long as the physicians cannot exactly define what they want, they will get what the vendors want them to get. The time has come to form a medical establishment powerful enough to set standards and thus communicate with the industrial partners as well as with the hospital managements responsible for purchasing. In fact a European project tries to specify such standards for PDMS, the EURISIC [44] project. Results should be presented in June 1994, at the European Congress of Intensive Care Medicine in Innsbruck, Austria.

At least it has to be mentioned, that the state of the art in PDMS is quite not satisfying at the moment. Still a lot of work has to be done to improve the performance, correct the defects and to fulfill the promises which have been given years ago. However, as long as the communication between the different partners is not improved too, the results will be poor: "For the science of medical informatics to be successful in achieving the primary goal of improving health care, it requires that the combined skills and knowledge of computer scientists, clinicians, nurses, paramedical professionals and researchers be brought together in a harmonious collaborative effort." [45]

9. Annotations and References

[1] Smith BE (1990) Universities and the clinical monitoring industry: Feckless independents or fruitful partners? Int J Clin Monitoring and Computing 7: 249–258

[2] Bowes CL, Ambroso C, Carson ER, Chambrin MC, Cramp D, Gilhooly K, et al (1992) INFORM: Development of information management and decision support systems for High Dependency Environments. Int J Clin Monitoring and Computing 8: 295–301

[3] Kalli S, Ambroso C, Gregory R, Heikelä A, Ilomäki A, Leaning M, et al (1992) Inform: Conceptual modelling of intensive care information systems. Int J Clin Monitoring and Computing 9: 85–94

[4] Groom DA, Harris JW (1990) Evaluation and selection of systems for automatic clinical operations. Biomedical Instrumentation & Technology May/June: 173–185

[5] Ambroso C, Bowes C, Chambrin MC, Gilhooly K, Green C, Kari A, et al (1992) INFORM: European survey of computers in Intensive Care Units. Int J Clin Monitoring and Computing 9: 53–61

[6] Leaning MS, Yates CE, Patterson DLH, Ambroso C, Collinson PO, Kalli ST (1991) A data model for intensive care. Int J Clin Monitoring and Computing 8: 213–224

[7] Shabot M (1989) Clinical systems as a focal point for distributed patient data. The Impact of Information Systems on Critical Care: A Look into the Future. Hewlett Packard, pp. 9–13

[8] Imhoff M, Piotrowski A, Reuß M (1992) Klinischer Einsatz eines Unix-basierten Klinischen Informationssystems für die Intensivmedizin. Biomedical Journal 34: 8–12

[9] See ref. [4]

[10] See ref. [6]

[11] Clinisoft

[12] GUI: Graphical User Interface, like MS Windows, or X-Windows or Apple's System 7

[13] If you are interested in that, contact e.g. Dr. Pollwein, Munich

[14] See also the paper of Martin et al. in this book

[15] MPEG: Motion Picture Expert Group; for further information see informatic issues, e.g.: Bertuch M (1993) Living bits on disc. CT, Magazin für Computer und Technologie 7: 118–120

[16] Nathe M (1992) Communication Standards. Proceeding of the 3rd Annual Meeting of the ESCTAIC, October 1992, p. X1

[17] Iaccobucci E (1989) Das OS/2 Buch. McGraw-Hill, New York

[18] LAN: Local Area Network

[19] See also chapter 4

[20] UPS: Uninterruptable Power Supply

[21] Paganelli BE (1989) Criteria for the Selection of a Beside Information System for Acute Care Units. Computers in Nursing 7: 214–221

[22] File server: a central computer in a network which holds the main-database

[23] Backup: copying your data to a (hopefully) secure place, e.g. an optical disc

[24] Graphical user interface for UNIX

[25] MT: Medical-Technical Devices

[26] This system provides limited possibility to display sections in graphic format: it is possible to configure six different screens with any combination of measured values

[27] In this system, all value displays are graphical displays

[28] No ventilators connected to this test-site until now

[29] To process medications, care-activities etc., you must buy the module I.N.C.A., which provides full PDMS-functionality in combination with the Atlantis system

[30] At entering a medication

[31] At entering a medication

[32] Usual in American systems: after selecting a care-diagnosis there is a set of care-activities automatically generated, a so called care-plan; it can be edited if needed

[33] Graphical display of the human body, which gives the nurses the possibility to select and mark different points with an input device, e.g. a mouse, and to describe the condition of the patient; this should simulate the situation as given in written documentation

[34] When producing a transfer report e.g.

[35] At this ward an external reporting-program was configured; if you don't have programming-engineers available it is recommendable to buy the module "Hospiprint", which acts as a print-server module. With this module you can configure any report you need

[36] With module Hospiimage

[37] But 24 -hours storage at HP-Merlin monitors; from there, the data can be taken

[38] Until the database becomes full; then the oldest patient data are deleted

[39] You can convert the ASCII-data-sets into any database

[40] These marks the possibility to display some valuable information during recording data; e.g. as you enter the prescribed cardiovascular medications, you would maybe like to see the trend of the HR and MAP of the last hours; systems with a "yes" have the ability to display such additional information in a window;

[41] I.N.C.A.: Integrated Nursing Care Applications

[42] CAREVUE, ATLANTIS and at the moment: CLINISOFT

[43] See also the paper of Wilding later in this book

[44] EURISIC: European Users Requirements for an Information System for Intensive Care

[45] Clemmer T, Gardner RM (1992) Medical informatics in the intensive care unit: State of the art 1991. Int J Clin Monitoring and Computing 8: 237–250

II. System Descriptions

EMTEK System 2000 – The Clinical Information Management System from Siemens

Siemens AG

Bereich Medizinische Technik, Erlangen, Germany

Hospitals today face major challenges:

- More acutely ill patients
- Increasing volumes of data and use of high-technology equipment
- Worldwide nursing shortage, particularly in the critical care field.

In this environment, hospitals have to make better use of resources and information. Nowhere is the opportunity for increasing staff productivity greater than in managing patient information.

The Idea

Emtek System 2000* is developed as a next-generation Clinical Information Management System to address hospitals' needs for automating the patient chart. The System 2000 puts an end to conventional handwritten documentation in the intensive care unit.

Up to now, critical care staff have relied on pen and paper to compile manual paper charts. Many nurses still use clipboards to record observations and measurements, even though the latter often come from automated sources. The time-consuming transcription of data on each patient does not always result in readable, or complete, data.

---

* The EMTEK System 2000 is designed and produced by EMTEK Health Care Systems, Inc., a subsidiary of Motorola Inc.; Siemens is the exclusive licensee for System 2000 in Europe

System 2000 provides accurate and up-to-date information, wherever it is needed.

The Solution

System 2000 places high-performance workstations, each with a large-screen display, keyboard and a mouse, at each bedside and in the doctor's office as well as at other central locations interconnected on a Local Area Network.

With automatic data acquisition from bedside instruments and pre-prepared lists for assessments, medications, physician orders and more, less time is spent for patient charting.

Even more important, however, are the following benefits:

— Repeated entries are not necessary; data need only enter the system once. Each intervention entered onto the flowsheet, for example, also appears in the status report.
— All patient documents are simultaneously available in the doctor's office, at the nurses' central station, as well as at every bedside.
— Lab data are automatically recorded.
— All interventions, both those prescribed and those actually performed, are thoroughly documented.
— Nurses can create complete care plans.
— All documents are always 100% up-to-date.
— All patient data are stored electronically and can be called up at any time for subsequent analysis.
— Peak work loads of the critical care staff can be detected and counteracted.
— And much more.

In order to achieve these benefits, familiar hospital forms are displayed on the screen. Paper, if used at all, serves only as a storage medium or for passing on information outside the ICU (for example, to non-automated units).

The Future

Intensive care units are the testing grounds for a Clinical Information Management System: System 2000 has long since passed all tests.

Ultimately, its open architecture and flexibility will be of use to nurses throughout the hospital.

Basic Characteristics

The thoracic operating room has different requirements for care and therapy than the neonatal ICU. Accordingly, the number, the format, and the contents of the System 2000 forms vary from hospital to hospital, ward to ward, discipline to discipline.

System 2000 offers the hospital a basic system which can be tailored to its special needs. Only a hospital-specific configuration can guarantee:

— Data display in an accepted format
— Efficient data acquisition which is tailored to the hospital and the application
— Trouble-free transition from manual charting to electronic charting.

Close contacts and continuous cooperation between the hospital and Siemens are prerequisites for the successful implementation of this Clinical Information Management System.

The process begins long before the hardware is delivered. Siemens systematically assists the hospital in a step-by-step implementation of the System 2000, which is thus customized to the special needs of each intensive care unit.

Forms

The electronic charts of System 2000 have the same look and feel as conventional handwritten charts. The displayed forms are based on the time-tested paper forms of the hospital. In this manner, for example, application-specific forms and/or treatment plans can be developed for specific illnesses.

In accordance with common clinical procedures, the same forms are used for both display and input of patient data. The critical care staff does not need to switch between a display mode and an entry mode.

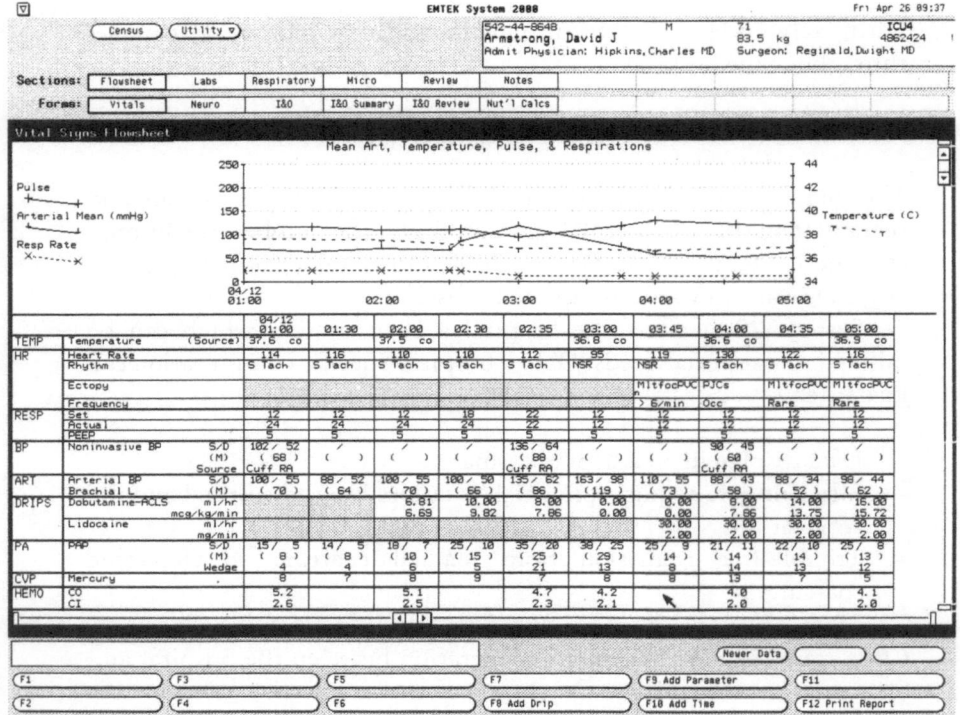

Fig. 1. The Vital Signs Flowsheet – complete, accurate, easy to use

After entry onto one form, data are automatically copy-forwarded to all applicable forms.

Related forms are grouped in sections which are predefined by the hospital.

Example:

Flowsheet	Assessments	Notes	Review	Lab	Care Planning
Flowsheet (vital signs)	Admission assessment	Important Status	Trend curves	Blood gas	Care plan
I/O	History	Treatments	Histograms	Hematology	Problem-
Electrolytes	Shift assess			Chemistry	list
Diet				Urine	Interventions
				Microbiology	

No more than two clicks of the mouse are needed to switch from one form to another.

Training

Typewriter skills or computer experience are not prerequisites for using this system. Even newcomers quickly master its use, thanks to an integrated help function and one simple principle: position the mouse, click the mouse.

Data Security

Generally, each patient's data are accessible from every workstation. However, System 2000 incorporates multi-level procedures for protecting patient data from unauthorized changes or viewing. Access rights to specific data or specific patients' data are restricted to authorized staff. All entries are stored with an associated signature to maintain a complete audit trail.

The incorporated security functions validate the electronic chart as a legal document.

Open Architecture

System 2000 is an open system in all respects. The hardware can be expanded at any time, without the need to replace existing equipment.

The software consists of program modules which can be combined – at any time – according to individual needs.

When the hospital is equipped with a Hospital Information System with centralized management of patients and beds, then admissions, transfers and discharges can all be processed from either the HIS or the System 2000 in the intensive care unit.

An interface to the lab computer system saves time and labor: authorized lab results are automatically sent to the corresponding forms of the System 2000.

Via the connection to a Picture Archiving and Communications System (PACS), digital X-ray images can be viewed at a System 2000 workstation – another time-saving feature for the decision-making process.

The staff's work load is also reduced by the automatic transfer of medication administration data and orders to the pharmacy computer.

Proven standard interfaces and communication protocols are currently available to various computer systems. Additional interfaces are in development.

Summary of the Most Important Functions

System 2000 manages all the information needed for the care and treatment of patients and puts this data in a useable format.

Assessment. Assessments document a patient's status from admission to discharge. These are compiled from context-sensitive lists and free-text entries. The current assessment is the basis for the care plan.

Care Planning. A library of standard care plans are already integrated in System 2000. For each assessment or problem case, a list of interventions and expected outcomes can be called up. These lists can be edited to provide patient-specific care plans.

Physician Orders. Hospital-specific order sets can be configured for medications, infusions, examinations, nutrition, etc. Using these lists and a mouse, orders can quickly be compiled without lengthy text entries. Verbal orders or orders via telephone can be entered later.

Task Lists. The system automatically generates patient-specific and shift-specific task lists on the basis of the hospital's standard procedures, the care plans, and the physician orders. These list the necessary interventions in chronological order.

When completed, tasks are checked off and disappear from the list. Corresponding forms are simultaneously updated. Interventions on ventilated patients appear in the ventilation chart, administered medications in the medication administration report, infusions in the I/O sheet, etc. Notes can be entered for uncompleted tasks.

Kardex. The Kardex documents all interventions which are prescribed and performed on a patient. Moreover, it can include other information such as the patient history, precautions, assessments, diet, allergies, etc. The Kardex is automatically administered by the system; only authorized staff can make corrections. Changes to the task list are automatically entered in the Kardex.

Vital signs. Vital signs are automatically acquired from connected bedside instruments and displayed in the corresponding patient charts. Interfaces are also available for acquisition of settings from ventilators and infusion pumps. Data can also be entered manually. At the touch of a key, derived parameters such as hemodynamic values are calculated and stored, using either standard or hospital-specific formulas.

Notes. Remarks, comments, and observations are important components of the patient chart and task lists; entries can be input or displayed at any time.

Lab Data. Lab data are acquired on-line from the laboratory computer system. Various interfaces are currently available. Even lab data on the patient before his/her admission to the unit are included. Special forms are also available for microbiology tests.

Intake and Output. The system calcualtes intake and output volumes for blood, fluids, and electrolytes, based on entries in the task list.

Printed Reports. All patient documentation can be printed, regularly or as needed, by high-speed laser printers.

Acuity. Special algorithms have been developed and parameters established to calculate acuity levels for severe injuries and high-risk patients. The goal: to determine adequate interventions.

System 2000 supports acuity scores and the severity index of Apache-II or other systems defined by the hospital.

Decision Support System. With the Decision Support System, all data of the System 2000 workstations are stored in a relational data base. Powerful tools make data query, analysis, and abstraction a reality, both during the patient's stay and after discharge. The on-line Decision Support System is suited to be the basis for future artificial intelligence systems.

Reliability

A system cannot fail in an intensive care unit. Such a system must be 100% available for several years. Stored data may not be lost. The unique design of System 2000 guarantees reliability.

System Architecture

The System 2000 workstations are some of the most powerful and reliable computers currently on the market.

All data on a patient are stored not only at the patient's bedside workstation, but also at at least one other workstation. This distributed

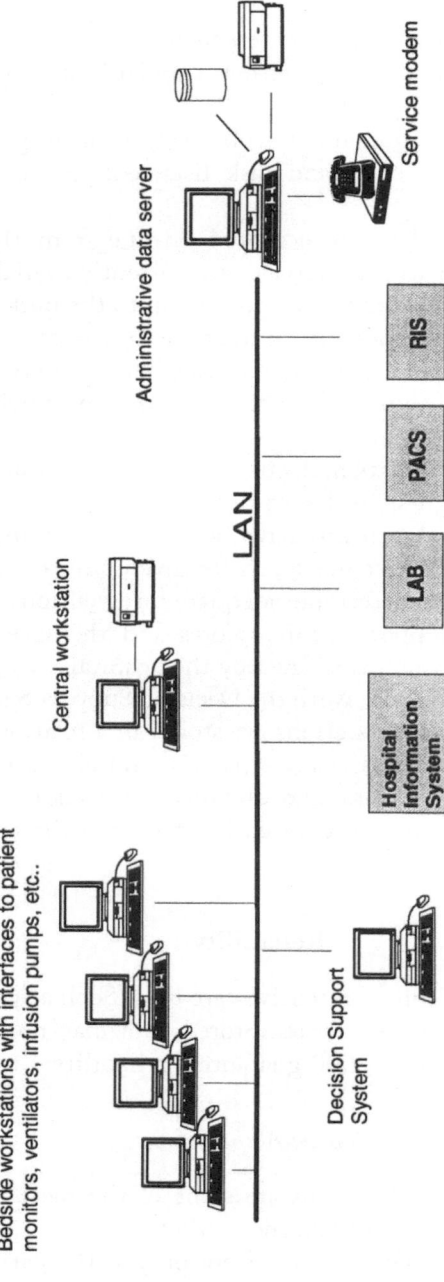

Fig. 2. System architecture

architecture means maximum data reliability, because patient data are retained and can be processed even in case of a complete failure of a workstation.

Software Quality

All System 2000 programs were developed and tested with the most modern equipment available. All functions run on a standard, unaltered UNIX operating system, whose reliability and flexibility have been proven a thousand times over.

Clinisoft – An Advanced Information System for the ICU

Clinisoft LTD

Kuopio, Finland

The ever growing flow of data increases the need for clerical work in intensive care. Therefore nurses have less time for the patient.

The quality of documentation changes paradoxically: during emergency the nurse has no time for record keeping – reconstructing the event is difficult.

The retrieval and assimilation of excessive amounts of data is difficult – the risk for omitting important information increases when short response time is critical.

The measures for quality assurance are time consuming or even impossible to perform with manual record keeping – no reliable information is available about quality of outcome or costs.

Clinisoft Information System Improves the Quality of Care

Automated data collection gives the nurses more time for patient care. The quality of documentation is independent of changes in the patient's clinical state – the system reliably and constantly reveals what is truly happening to the patient. Decisions based on relevant information promote patient safety and quality of care.

The system assists actively in the planning and execution of therapy by *context specific presentation* technique: data associated to an individual decision or intervention is displayed to help decison making. No more cumbersome wandering through complicated menu structures.

The system is *extremely configurable:* most of its functions can be configured by the user without any programming skills. Even the default orders for care and examinations can be defined according to an individual ICU and the patient group. These care protocols markedly enhance the planning of care in most cases.

The system provides efficient tools for *quality assurance* both in nursing care and medical treatment. It helps in daily resource management and in the long term planning of the department.

The system is independent of the types of bedside instruments in use. It can be adapted to all ICU environments.

Product Architecture

Clinisoft Information System for intensive care is a distributed microcomputer system. It consists of three types of workstations:

- bedside workstations
- office workstations
- servers

The bedside workstations take care of the automatic data collection from patient devices. The bedside workstations also act as nurses' workstations for input of manual data and displays for therapy orders and data trends. The devices are connected to a bedside workstation via a connection panel.

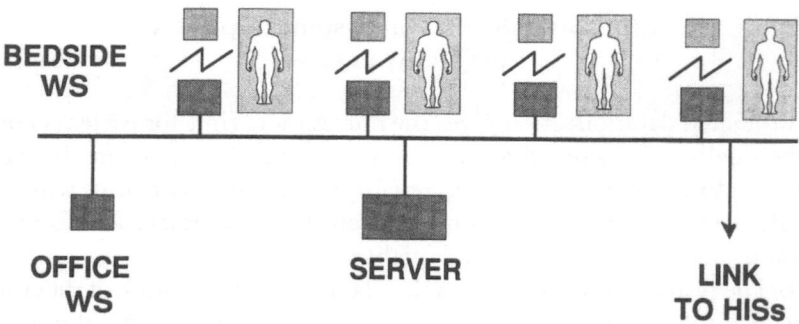

Fig. 1

All patient data can be reviewed and therapy planned at the office workstations. They are also used for patient administration (admission, discharge etc.).

The system follows the client-server architecture. All data is stored in the server's database.

General Features

Clinisoft Information System for Intensive Care supports patient and unit management. Patient-related tasks are both clinical and administrative while unit-related functions contain short-term and long-term operations, e.g. staff management and statistical follow-ups.

The bedside workstation approach ensures data collection and enhances the use of information. All information is accessed quickly and efficiently from all workstations.

The system is easy to learn. The screens and functions are designed according to graphical user interface standards. There are multiple ways to move within the system and access the functions.

The system is delivered with desired language. A build-in help facility is always available. In addition Clinisoft will train clinical users and support the use continuously.

Simple but effective forms of decision aids are included in the system. The use of associative data presentation focuses the user's attention into essential information. Patient group related default orders and records will decrease the amount of human errors and speed up the use of the system.

Patient Administration

Operations supporting patient administration contain admission, discharge, temporary discharge and bedplace changes. Diagnoses and surgical operations are recorded by using a desired coding system. Reports can be printed out and also redesigned according to local needs.

Medication

The planning of medication can be assisted by user defined associative displays, which present for example the trends of serum digoxin and creatinine concentrations when digoxin is chosen from the drug list. User defined defaults enhance the prescription of the dose, route and duration of the medication.

The past history of the medications can be easily and comprehensively displayed when necessary.

The system supports in carrying out the drug therapy by collecting all prescriptions to the nurse's task list and providing the nurse with an efficient pump organiser for drug infusions.

Fluid Therapy

The fluid therapy option is divided into the maintenance and replacement parts, which helps to organize the fluid therapy plan properly. Replacement orders can be effectively linked with cardiovascular management.

The use of predefined default fluid therapy programs for the patient groups reduces the need of repeated keyboard operations.

Automatic retrieval of data from infusion pumps makes it possible to provide the user with updated input-output data, which makes it easier to achieve the aimed 24 hour input-output balance.

The infusion display helps the nurse to assign the prescribed fluids to the pumps. Fluids to be given without a pump can also be included in the plan.

Respiratory Care

Monitoring and planning of respiratory care is efficiently supported from chest physiotherapy to the most complicated cases of ventilatory support.

The displays for planning the respiratory care and for the documentation of care given adapt automatically to the chosen type of ventilator.

Automatic data collection from computer interfaced ventilators dramatically reduce the clerical work of the nurses and increase the quality of documentation.

Care Plan

Care plan assists in rationale planning and assesment of patient care. It's a tool both for nurses and physicians. The use of care plan creates a functional link between planning and administration of care. Nursing care protocols can be activated with care plan. Patient's current state is summarized in care plan which improves shift to shift information change between care providers.

Graphics

Data about observations and nursing tasks are entered by using a graphic human figure. For example, information about an inserted catheter is entered by pointing its location on the human graph. Details are entered through a form window. The information can be accessed again by clicking the symbol on the graph.

Graphics are used throughout the system. Trend figures, colours and human graphs replace traditional text-form expressions. Tiny

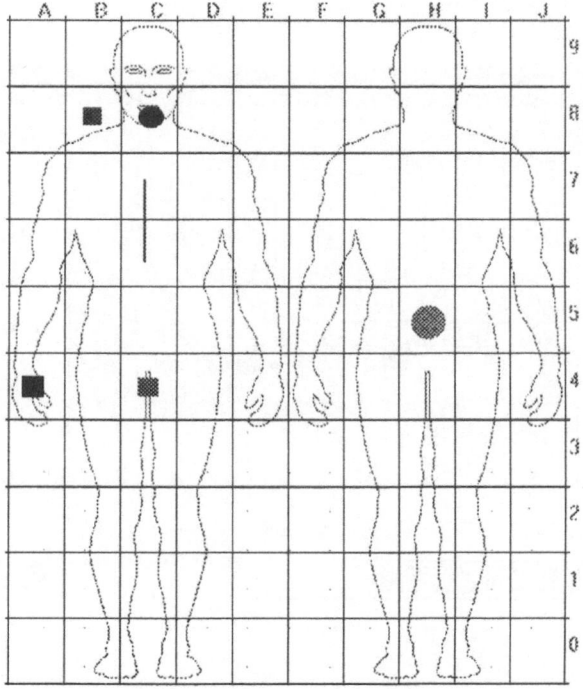

Fig. 2

picture symbols (icons) are used to facilitate selections and to indicate that related information is available. Generally, clicking an icon reveals more detailed information or initiates a function.

Trends

Monitored data is automatically fed in by using connections to monitors and other bedside devices. Information provided by these devices is displayed as numeric arrays and graphic trend figures. Trend pages can be easily designed to provide the unit with a graphic expression of any recorded variable – monitored data, laboratory results and observations.

Graphic trend presentation supports the assessment of patient state and the effect of therapy.

Both time and value scales can be altered while using a trend display.

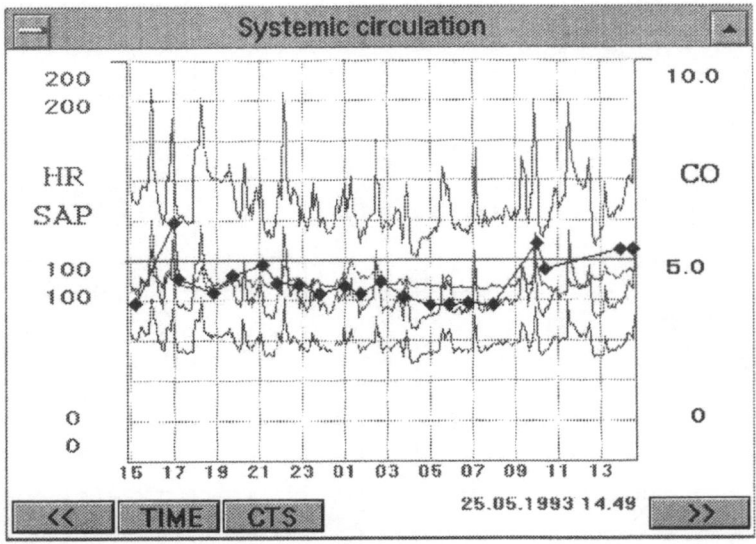

Fig. 3

Task List

The task list helps nurses to organise their daily work. All new prescriptions are automatically added in the task list. The nurse can use the list as a memorandum by entering new tasks herself. When a task has been completed, it can be confirmed in the task list. If a task has not been completed in a predefined time the system triggers an alert signal.

Laboratory

The system can be connected to the hospital's laboratory information system to send requests and to receive results directly back to the system. Routine request sets can be designed according to patient grouping to speed up ordering process. Laboratory results can be presented both in numeric and graphic format.

Connection to Bedside Devices

Devices with a computer interface can be connected into the system. This feature allows automatic data collection from patient monitors, oxymeters, ventilators and infusion pumps.

    As far as the electric connections are concerned, special attention has been paid to patient safety. Automatic data collection increases speed and accuracy, and saved time can be used for other tasks in patient care. Critical situations when the personnel is occupied in emergency care do not interrupt documentation of monitored data.

Short-Term Unit Management

Patient list displays all bedplaces, giving an overview of the current situation in the unit. Clicking a bed on the map reveals more information on the patient.

    The short-term unit management includes also resource management such as inventory, personnel and bedside devices. Invoicing can be configured according to local needs.

HOSPITAL					DEMOGRAPHY					
Intensive care unit					10.06.93					

ICU STAYS 01.01.92 - 31.03.93

Diagn group	Type	Stays	Days	Length	APACHE II	TISSavg	TISStot	TISS/ APACHE	Mort/icu %	Aort/hosp %
1000	elec	8	25,0	3,1	20	17	425	0,9	0,0	0,0
1000	emer	94	344,5	3,7	20	35	12 144	1,8	2,2	4,3
1100	elec	15	51,0	3,4	16	24	1 224	1,5	0,0	

Fig. 4

Long-Term Unit Management

The long-term unit management includes a comprehensive reporting facility. The system has also a spreadsheet calculation interface. Using it the management can create needed unit spesific reports.

The facility for correlating detailed information of costs with standard severity and intensivity measures may significantly influence on the long-term cost-benefit ratio of the unit.

Help

Information on using the system can always be recalled in a help window. As default, information on functions of the current active display is provided. A comprehensive help index is included in the help function.

Care Manuals

Various instructions and operating manuals can be typed into the system. They can then be accessed via any workstation by using keywords and indexes. This feature replaces traditional paper files and always provides the reader with up-to-date information.

Clinisoft for Efficient ICU Management

Clinisoft assists planning, allocation of resources, follow-up, quality assurance and cost accounting in the intensive care unit. Comprehensive reporting produces up-to-date information for the unit management.

Care Planning and Documentation
with the Patient Data Management System (PDMS)
CareVue 9000

H. Vedovelli, MD

Hewlett Packard Medical Systems Group, Vienna, Austria

Summary

In the Critical Care environment the utilization of computer aided care plans in combination with work lists and an electronic flowsheet increases quality of patient care and documentation. Eight ICUs in two large hospitals in Vienna using a PDMS for more than one year have gathered experience with electronic charting at the bedside. HP Care-Vue 9000 is able to support the care process providing tools that are replacing paper based documentation. In addition, care research can be performed with statistical tools.

Introduction

Since the beginning of the nineties, a broad use of bedside computers for patient documentation in the critical care environment has been implemented for the first time. In the Allgemeines Krankenhaus (AKH) Vienna and the Donauspital (SMZ) Vienna there are now eight systems of the type Hewlett Packard CareVue 9000 in use for daily charting at Medical and Anesthesiological ICU's. The first systems have been in use now for over one year. Daily use has shown that a major part of the documentation is done by the nursing staff. According to this fact, one of the main goals of the software design for such a system is the support of the nurse care plans and documentation.

Hardware and Software

The PDMS HP CareVue 9000 is a system of bedside Apollo workstations based on Motorola's 68040 processor or HP PA-RISC (Precision Architecture – Reduced Instruction Set Computing). The application software runs under the multi-user, multi-tasking operating system HP-UX.

Requests

Among the different requests for a PDMS as online-data transfer from bedside medical-technical devices, communication with other systems, data export and security, a main issue for the care process is the structure of the software. Here, the following issues are of importance:

- Support of the care process from planning to documentation
- Easy to use
- Standardization of the documentation for quality assurance
- Therefore, scientific evaluation of routine charted data later on.

Software Design

The HP CareVue 9000 Application software is based on a model that simulates the daily bedside care process (Fig. 1). Each step of the care process is implemented in a module. The integration of the different modules leads the user through the application. A part of the modules described below are in use today; with the following two updates of the software the system will be completed.

The first step of the documentation begins with the nursing assessment, which consists in HP CareVue 9000 of a set of configurable categories that can be configured to meet the needs of each specific ICU. Based on this nursing assessment, the system creates a first care plan. Here, the nurse has the choice to select from a configurable list of standard care plans or configurable single steps. The system puts all the steps of the first care plan into a worklist.

Each step of the care process appears twice: once in a problem oriented view on the care plan, once time oriented on the worklist.

With progress notes, the nurse can evaluate the care plan in order to be able to check it for an expected outcome. Changes of

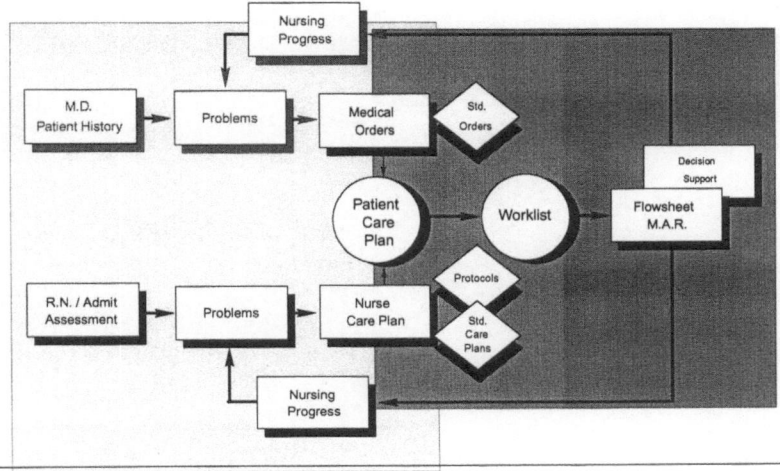

Fig. 1

treatments and therapy are automatically updated in the care plan and worklist.

Ergonomic data entry is important for a computer system in the clinical environment. This is supported by a trackball with preconfigured choice lists and structured text in order to minimize the use of the keyboard to entry of text.

The use of preconfigured choice lists and structured text is also useful for the continuity of the documentation and for data evaluation. As a side effect, the flowsheets are always legible by those who have a password. These functions should improve the quality of documentation.

With the possibility of computer aided data evaluation on an additional statistical computer, care research can be supported as well.

Conclusion

With the use of a computer aided patient care plan linked to a resulting worklist, the care process can be structured and made more efficient.

Experiences with a PC-Based Indifferent Communicating PDM-System

T. Neugebauer, M. Hiesmayr, E. Donner, D. Heilinger, P. Keznickl,
P. Mares, W. Zwölfer, and W. Haider

Department of Cardiothoracic Anaesthesia and Intensive Care Medicine,
Research Institute for Intensive Care Medicine, Vienna, Austria

Abstract

In the year 1991 the Research Departement for Intensive Therapy at
the University School of Medicine in Vienna installed the Patient Data
Management (PDM) system 'ATLANTIS' from 'HUMAN MICRO-
PROCESSING' (hmp), 'HOSPITRONICS', at two Intensive Care
Units (cardiothoracic and mixed surgical and general).

Since this semigraphical version was used largely successfully, it
was replaced by the new full graphical version ATLANTIS-GUI
(Graphical User Interface) in March 1993. The first practical experiences of this version are presented.

The main characteristics of the system ATLANTIS are the use of
network connected standard IBM PCs and the ability of the system to
communicate indifferently with any medico-technical device, independently from its manufacturer. The only condition is a standard
serial port (RS232) on the device. Therefore within the short time of
some weeks the patient monitors, the ventilators, the pulsoxymeters
and the perfusion pumps have been successfully connected to the
system.

One of the most important advantages of a PC system is the fact
that it is an open system. For this reason a lot of programs, developed
by the users of the system, could be integrated. These are for example
programs for transfer of the results of the main laboratory and of the

local acute laboratory, furthermore a program for 24 hours summary printouts, adapted to the requests of the ward. This open architecture, together with the use of DESQview, allows the use of other programs that share data with the PDM, for example a program for computer-assisted weaning from the ventilator (KBWEAN). A program for communication with the host system of the scientific computer center of the university is under development. With this communication it will be possible to use the data base and of the complete statistical tools of the scientific computer center.

Another important advantage of a PC system are the high performance and speed at the local workstation. As the computing and memory capacities and the device communication are distributed in a PC network, the performance at the local workstation is not dependent from the number of workstations. In the full graphical version of ATLANTIS it lasts only for some parts of a second in most cases to open a new window.

In the semigraphical version there had been some defects, most of them have been eliminated in the new full graphical version, a lot of details had been improved considerably.

In conclusion, the concept of a PDM system, based on PCs in a network and of indifferent communication at the bedside, can be regarded as a practical and approved solution with a potential of multiple uses. In the daily clinical work the presentation of trends of various parameters, simultaneously to the actual monitoring, proved to be a great benefit. It can be expected, that this system, together with the module for care planning and documentation which is now under installation, may allow the change to mainly electronic bedside documentation in the near future.

Introduction

Beginning with midth of 1991, the Research Departement for Intensive Therapy at the University School of Medicine in Vienna installed and extended step by step the Patient Data Management (PDM) system 'ATLANTIS' from 'HUMAN MICROPROCESSING' (hmp), 'HOSPITRONICS', at two Intensive Care Units (cardiothoracic and mixed surgical and general). Since this semigraphical version was used largely successfully, it is going to be replaced by the new full graphical version ATLANTIS-GUI (Graphical User Interface) since March 1993. The first practical experiences of the users with this version are presented.

The main characteristics of the system ATLANTIS are, on the one hand, the use of IBM Token Ring network connected standard IBM PCs with the MS-DOS operating system. Beside the economical advantage, compared with other operating systems (e.g. UNIX), the greatest benefit of a DOS system is the fact, that it is an open system. You can use a lot of well known PC programs for different applications and analyses, furthermore, programs developed by the users themselves can be integrated easily. These programs can share the datas of the PDM. This advantage is very important especially in an university hospital.

On the other hand, the ability of the system to communicate indifferently with any medico-technical device, independently from its manufacturer, is the second great advantage. The only condition is a standard serial port (RS232) on the device.

The System

The Installation

The Personal Computers are IMB PS/2 Modell 70-A21 PCs, containing an 80386 processor with a clock frequency of 25 MHz, a floating point processor 80387, a memory capacity of 8 MB and a hard disk of 120 MB. The operating system is DOS 5.0. To run the ATLANTIS software, you need DESQview V2.4 for multi tasking and the expanded memory manager QEMM-386 V6.0, both from Quarterdeck. The built in serial port and a multiport card with 8 additional serial ports are used for communication with the medico-technical devices at the bedside. At the PCs at the bedside you find ergonomically designed track balls ('TRACKMAN' from LOGITECH).

The PCs are connected in an IBM Token Ring Local Area Network (LAN) with Typ 1 cables and Novell 3.11 of NetWare as network software. In our case an important advantage of the IBM Token Ring comes from the fact, that the IBM Token Ring is the standard network technology of the Institut of Medical Computer-Sciences (IMC) in the new building of the hospital. Therefore the hardware connection to the mainframe of the IMC is not really a problem and is under realisation.

There is a PC at each of the 24 beds in two Intensive Care Units (ICUs) and additionally in both the doctors and the nurses rooms in the two units, in the local acute laboratory and in the technician's room. In this room there are also the file seNer (an IBM PS/2 Modell 80-A31 with 8 MB memory and an 320 MB hard disk), an optical disk station for permanent data storage, a PC for network administration and three PCs for communication. In both ICUs there is duplex Laser Printer (Hewlett Packard LaserJet 111 D). Particularly emphasized should be the fact that, for the present, in one cardiothoracic surgery room a PC for anesthesia documentation is connected. Therefore it is possible to get continuous documentation of automatically collected patient datas from the operating room and the ICU in one system. The only interruption is the transport time. Finally there is a PC connected to the LAN in the laboratory of the operating theatre.

The Bedside Communication

The communication of the PCs with the medico-technical devices at the bedside is a standard serial communication via the RS232. At present at each bed a haemodynamic patient monitor 'HORIZON 2000' of MENNEN MEDICAL, a ventilator 'Evita' of DRAEGER and a pulsoxy- and capnometer 'OSCAR' of DATEX are integrated. The transmitted parameters are the heart rate, up to four invasive blood pressures, pulmonary wedge pressure and cardiac output, the respiratory frequency, two temperatures, a lot of venti-lation parameter settings and measured values (Venvmin, FiO_2, TVexp, PIP, PEEP, ...), the pulsoxymetric oxygen saturation (SpO_2) and the end-expiratory CO_2. Via the interface 'DIANET' of BRAUN, up to six perfusion pumps 'PERFUSOR SECURA FT' of BRAUN can be connected. The settings of the flow rate are transmitted.

The Personal Computer in the cardio thoracic operating room communicates with a monitoring device of HELLIGE, with the anesthesia machine 'Cicero' of DRAEGER an with the pulsoxy- and capnometer 'OCSAR OXY' of DATEX.

The online transmitted datas of the different bedside devices and of the acute laboratory are stored automatically in a time interval of 1 to 60 minutes. At present the default interval is set to 10 minutes. As the datas are stored both on the local hard disk and on the hard disk of the file server, the data security is present.

The software part for data acquisition is a special module called HMIB (Human Micro-processing Medical Information Bus). It is running in a DESQview window, largely independently from the module for data storage and presentation. Datas, transmitted to the system via the file server (e.g. laboratory datas), are also taken over by the HMIB module.

The Data Presentation

The automatically stored values are presented in tables for different types of parameters (haemodynamic, respiratory and laboratory parameters, medications and fluids), additional in various graphics. The order and the label of the parameters in the tables are configurable, so are the number and the kind of parameters, the colors, symbols and kind of presentation and the titles in the graphics. The fluid input, output and the balance are presented in a clear bar graph (cf. Fig.1). By selecting a point with the mouse curser in a graphic, the values of the most important parameters and comments at this point of time are listed on the screen.

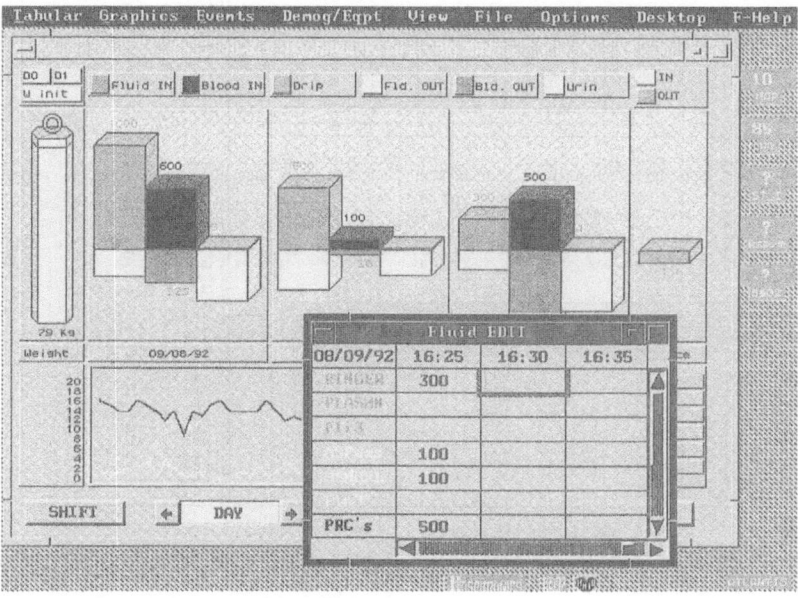

Fig. 1. Example of a bar graph of the fluid balance

T. Neugebauer et al.

The Laboratory Communication

The system gets laboratory results automatically both from the main laboratory of the clinical departement and from the local acute laboratory in the ICU. For the communi-cation with main laboratory its computer, an IBM RISC 6000, was directly connected to the IBM Token Ring. A program, developed in the 'Research Departement for Intensive Therapy', takes over the laboratory results from this compu-

---

Herzchirurgische Instensivstation - B200
Leiter: Univ. Prof. Dr. W. Haider
Tel:40400/2343   Fax:40400/2331

Seite 1

Forschungsstelle für Intensivtherapie

Patient: Berger   Bett: 12   Tag: 28/12/92

Cardiovascular Data

Date	28/12	28/12	28/12	28/12	28/12	28/12	28/12	29/12	29/12	29/12	29/12	29/12
Time	08-10	10-12	12-14	14-16	16-18	18-20	20-22	22-24	00-02	02-04	04-06	06-08
HR	103	118	103	102	102	118	109	105	114	124	129	124
SPa	102	111	117	111	115	113	115	120	120	101	96	109
DPa	46	53	58	58	60	62	63	63	61	51	47	54
MAP	65	71	75	74	76	78	79	80	79	68	65	72
CVP												
CO												
SPp	43	46	53	52	53	46	48	49	45	41	40	41
DPp	24	25	25	27	16	25	28	27	24	24	24	24
MPA	32	34	36	37	30	34	36	36	33	31	31	31
LAM	16	17	16	16	16	15	19	17	15	13	13	14
PCWP	13											
TMP1												
TMP2												

Respiratory Data

Date	28/12	28/12	28/12	28/12	28/12	28/12	28/12	29/12	29/12	29/12	29/12	29/12
Time	08-10	10-12	12-14	14-16	16-18	18-20	20-22	22-24	00-02	02-04	04-06	06-08
Rsp/m	14	15	14	7	5	7	9	9	14	14	14	14
EtCO2	32.9	40.8	45.6	10.4	3.3	21.7	27.0	33.9	36.8	35.5	36.3	35.9
SaO2	63.5	84.0	87.8	83.1	92.8	91.1	70.1	77.7	95.8	95.6	95.6	96.4

Ventilatory Data

Date	28/12	28/12	28/12	28/12	28/12	28/12	28/12	29/12	29/12	29/12	29/12	29/12
Time	08-10	10-12	12-14	14-16	16-18	18-20	20-22	22-24	00-02	02-04	04-06	06-08
Fio2	52	52	51	51	51	51	51	51	51	51	51	52
PIP	28	28	26	25	24	25	25	25	25	25	25	25
PEEP	15	15	12	12	9	9	9	9	9	9	9	9
Pmean	15	15	14	15	15	15	15	14	15	15	15	15
TVle	1151	1009	999	1019	1062	1036	955	1058	1159	1109	1067	965
MinVol	20	17	18	19	22	20	21	19	17	17	18	19
I:E												
Vrate												

Astrup Data

Date	28/12	28/12	28/12
Time	16:31	18:01	23:31
pHa	7.37	7.37	7.421
pCO2a	50.6	52	45.1
pO2a	139	101	120
Sat_A	98.2	97.2	98.1
Sat_V	79.9		
Bi/BE	3.7	4.4	5
Hgb	11.5	11.3	10.2
Na+	132	131	132
K+	4.9	4.6	4.2
Glu	141	132	128

Laboratory Data

	Date 28/12/92
	Time 08:00
Leuko	4.6
Ery	* 3.59
Hb	* 10.3
HK	* 30.9
Thromb	* 89
PTZ	67
PTT	---
RZ	* 29.1
Fibr.	* 726
AT III	* 67
TZ	* 28.3
Na	* 134
K	4.40
Cl	* 94
BUN	* 55.2
Ca	* 2.07
Mg	0.94
an. P	1.38
HS	---
Gluc.	* 119
TRIGLY	142
CHOL	* 70
S.Bili	* 2.78
B.dir.	* 2.7
NH3	---
LAKT	* 2.2
a-AMYL	---
P.AMYL	---
LIPASE	---
AP	* 293
GOT	10
GPT	3
g-GT	* 34
LDH	* 274
a-HBDH	---
CK	15
CK-MB	---
Fr. Hb	---
GEW	* 4.8
DIGOX	---
DIGITO	* 12.04
CHINID	---
GENTA	---
VANCO	* 9.75
CYMO	---
H.Na	* 32
H.K	38
H.BUN	* 412
H.Krea	* 41
H.EW	---
H.Amyl	---

Comments:

Fig. 2 a

Fig. 2 a, b. Example of the daily 24 hours printouts developed by the users

ter with a standard PC-Host-Protocoll ('PC/TCP'), adapts the data format to the requirements of the ATLANTIS software and writes the values in a file on the file server hard disk. The HMIB module reads the values from this file.

The programs for the communication with the blood gas analyser IL 1306 in the local acute laboratory and with the blood gas analyser BGE in the laboratory of the operating theatre, both devices of 'Instrumentation Laboratory', were developed also in the 'Research Departement for Intensive Therapy'. Besides this online communication you can make corrections or add some values by hand.

The Printouts

The standard ATLANTIS printouts did not meet the requirements of the stations completely. You cannot select a different time scale for the

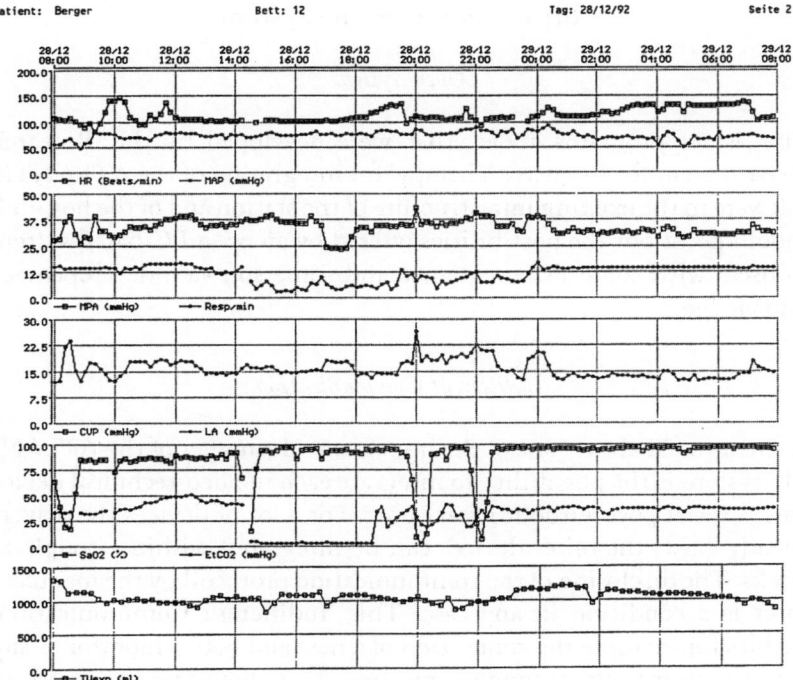

Fig. 2 b

tables and the graphics in one printout for example. This causes a lot of paper with tables when you are interested in a detailed resolution of the graphics only. Therefore the 'Research Departement for Intensive Therapy' developed a software for printing a 24 hours protocoll on one double-page (size A4), adapted to the special requirements of the stations. This program can be started from a LAN connected printer PC and reads the actual datas of the patients from the hard disk of the file server. There is an example of the printouts in Figs. 2 a, b.

The Storage of the Datas When you exit the ATLANTIS program, the user has to decide whether he wants the datas to be stored permanently or to be given free for being overwritten by the datas of the next patient. In case of an error in that selection you could lose important datas. The 'Research Departement for Intensive Therapy' developed a small program for automatic permanent strorage of all the raw datas on an optical disc in any case.

Strong Points of the System

Open System

The list of programs above, that were developed by the 'Research Departement for Intensive Therapy' for integration of the ATLANTIS software in the existing infrastructure of the station and of the hospital, should point out the possibilities offered by an open PC-based system to users with some PC experience and some software developement knowledge.

Indifferent Communication

As mentioned above, one of the important advantages of the ATLAN-TIS system is the possibility to integrate each medico-technical device with a serial port without great effort. For a lot of devices the drivers already exist, the other devices can be integrated within a couple of weeks. The disclosing of the communication protocoll by the manufacturer is a condition in any case. This 'Indifferent Communication' enables for example the connection of a new and better monitor of any manufacturer to the system at any time. This should be an important aspect, especially in an university hospital.

Multi Tasking

The multi tasking user interface DESQview 2.40 makes it possible to run the PDM-System ATLANTIS and other DOS applications at one PC simultaneously. An example of such a program, that moreover reads the actual ATLANTIS datas, is the expert system 'KBWEAN'. That program, which was developed together with the IMC, is described in an other article in that book. It makes suggestions for the optimisation of the weaning from the ventilator on the base of flexible rules, applied to the actual datas of a patient.

IMC-Communication

A program for communication with the host system of the Institute for Medical Computer-Sciences (IMC), the scientific computer center of the university, is under development. With this communication it will be possible to transmit datas to the data base system 'WAREL' and make use of the complete statistical tools of the SAS. As the technology of the local PC network and the network of the IMC in the new building of the hospital is an IBM Token Ring in both cases, the hardware connection of the LAN to the mainframe of the IMC is not a great problem and is under realisation.

High Performance

Other important advantages of a PC system are the high performance and speed at the local workstation. As the computing and memory capacities and the device communication are distributed in a PC network, the performance at the local PC-workstation is not influenced even through a large number of beds respectively PC-workstations. In the full graphical version ATLANTIS-GUI it lasts only for some parts of a second to open or switch to a new window in most cases.

Weak Points of the System

Weak Points of the Software

There had been some defects in the semigraphical version of ATLAN-TIS, most of them have been eliminated and a lot of details had been improved considerably in the new full graphical version ATLANTIS-GUI. So the tables and graphics are farely configurable now. We still miss the possibility to structure the tables to get a better and faster overview. Further it is not possible to show one parameter in different tables at the same time. In contrast to the semigraphical version the graphics have no scaling grid, therefore the association of a certain point of a graph to a value or a time is not as fast and easy as it was. Also missing in the new version is the continuation of the flow rates of the perfusion pumps put in by hand.

The lack of configurability of the daily printouts could be overcome by a user developed software as described above.

The system has still no integrated patient and bed administration for the ICU, an user developed software could be a solution in this point too.

The communication with the connected bedside medico-technical devices (monitor, ventilator, pulsoxy- and capnometer) and the transfer of laboratory datas from the file server is working without any problems in most cases, some problems in certain points still yet exist. So the Cardiac Output and the Pulmonary Wedge Pressure are not taken over from the monitor in many cases, and the driver for communication with the perfusion pumps of BRAUN via the DIANET interface still needs some changings for a practicable pump to drug association.

Finally should be mentioned, that the expectantion we had in the system at the beginning, that it should be possible to develope device drivers by ourselves, has not been met up to now in spite of promises by the manufacturer. The reason therefore might be lack of information or just a different setting of priorities on our part up to now. That would be a very interesting aspect for an flexible university system anyway, you could integrate new devices just for testing by yourself.

Weak Points of the Hardware

The only system problem determined by the hardware occured up to now is the textile dust sucked in by the ventilator of the PCs. In declared medico-technical devices with a ventilator this problem also occures, but it is mostly solved in a better way than it is in a standard PC. The ventilation slits are covered with a some millimeter thick layer of textile dust after half a year of running, the floopy disk drives have to be cleaned before usage in most cases. These drives, however, are nearly never used on the one side, on the other side they can be protected with a simple adhesive tape. Apart from this the dust did not cause severe problems until now, a periodical inside cleaning of the PCs seems to be recommended anyway.

Conclusion

The question which is probably the most important one is that for the benefit for the patients of such a system. From our experiences up to now we can say, that the continuous graphical presentation of the trends of various vital parameters of the last hours, simultaneously and additionally to the actual monitoring, proved to be a great benefit. Critical developements of the patient's state can be recognized earlier. Another benefit is the availability of results of the local acute laboratory and of the main laboratory immediately after analysis directly at the patient's bed, frequentely hours before you get the printed comprehensive report.

The evaluation of clinical studies with datas of automatic periodic data acquisition enables clearer results than studies with datas irregularly protocolled by hand in many cases. A new matter are programs like the expert system for computerassisted optimisation of the weaning process from the ventilator mentioned above. First practical tests are very encouraging. The possibility to have other programs running at the bedside that share the PDM system's data further allows the developement of 'Smart Alarm Systems' with integrated data interpretation and simultaneous evaluation of trends in different variables.

Integration of Patient Monitors into a Data Management System for the Intensive Care Unit

J. Martin[1], J. Hiller[2], M. Messelken[1], and P. Milewski[1]

[1] Clinic for Anesthesiology, Intensive Care Medicine and Pain Therapy,
[2] Department of Medicine Technology,
Klinik am Eichert, Göppingen, Germany

Abstract

A large number of therapy-relevant decisions in intensive care medicine touch upon the results of clinical examinations and investigations from several different sources. A computer supported system that gathers and evaluates these results is now available and in the future it appears that such a system will be indispensable. The following pages will describe a data management system that ties together patient bedside monitors with laboratory parameters, work lists and other types of information. The data management system then makes this information available at the patient's bedside without having to place a second workstation terminal at the bedside. Vital sign parameters are concurrently collected on-line and can be stored or printed at a central workstation.

Information processing is optimized through this inexpensive integration of patient monitors into a data management system for the intensive care unit. Physicians are then able to more quickly reach a decision regarding therapy. At the same time, it can also be shown that the system can relieve some of the burdens carried by the physician and nursing staff.

Introduction

Modern intensive care medicine is increasingly dependent on productive communications and information technologies [6]. The numerous external and internal clinical findings must be brought together so that it is possible to make a meaningful decision about therapy. The demand that all therapy relevant clinical findings must be available at the bedside is quite difficult to realize without a computer supported system. The ideal solution would be to have a second workstation terminal next to the patient monitor which replaces the trend curves [2]. A few systems which meet these conditions are currently offered by industry. Nevertheless, such a system cannot be installed in every intensive care unit due to the lack of sufficient space or because of the scarcity of funds.

There are currently new systems available that tie patient monitors into a single data management system. The advantage of such a system is that no additional space at the bedside is required, and the personnel, who are already familiar with the use of patient monitors, do not need a significant amount of training in order to be able to use and understand the new functions offered by such a system.

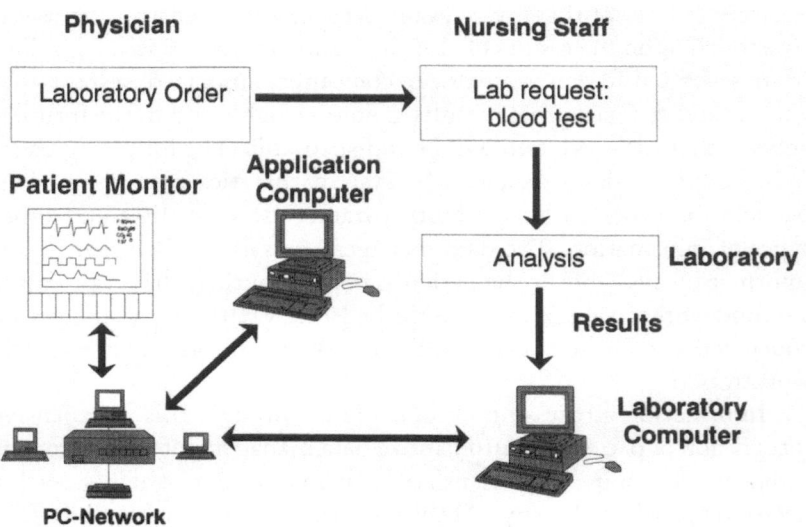

Fig. 1. Lab request and on-line lab data transfer to the bedside patient monitors

One or two computer workstations can acquire the necessary patient data without a problem. By connecting the computer workstation into a PC network, which can itself be linked to a laboratory workstation, important information is made available, which supports an expeditious decision making process. At the same time, some of the work burden of the medical staff is removed due to the fact that the collection of clinical findings is no longer applicable.

Through the graphical user interface of the workstation and through the integration of the data management system with the familiar functionality of the patient bedside monitors, personnel quickly learn how to use the system thereby leading to a high level of acceptance [2] (Fig. 1).

Hardware

The 12 bed intensive care unit is equipped with the modular Component Monitoring System (CMS) patient monitors from the Hewlett-Packard Company. In order to attain a comprehensive view of the alarms in the ICU, the patient monitors are connected to the Serial Distribution Network (SDN).

The computer workstations are PC compatible computers with a 386 processor at a 25 MHz clockrate. Other components include an 80 megabyte (MB) hard disk and 12 MB random access memory (RAM). The server on the PC network is a 486/25 PC with 16 MB RAM and a hard disk with a capacity of 1 gigabyte. The gateway between the laboratory's UNIX based central computer and the PC network is a 386 laptop computer with 4 MB of RAM and a 40 MB hard disk.

Standard Software

The operating system of the server and application computers is OS/2 version 1.3. Microsoft LAN Manager 2.1 was installed as the network software. The remaining client workstations that are connected to the network run the MS-DOS operating system version 5.0.

Step-By-Step Description of the System

After the patient has been admitted to the intensive care unit, he or she is connected to the patient monitor. By pressing a simple combination of function keys on the patient monitor, a "Fast Admission" of the patient can be carried out. With this type of admission the patient is assigned a unique identification number by the system and registration of the on-line vital sign parameters begins.

Before the system can begin sending information like Lab Data, worklists and other medical information to the patient bedside monitor, the patient must fully be admitted within the software application. This must be done at one of the application workstations. The reason for this is that only by using unambiguous identification, for instance the patient admission number, is it possible to have a secure, bedside allocation of Lab Data and other clinical findings.

Should the patient be transferred within the intensive care unit, the transfer can be carried out either at the bedside by using a selection list at the patient monitor, or within the software application at the central workstation. Also, a re-admission for the continuation of data acquisition of trend curves and other wave forms of a patient is possible by utilizing the selection list at the patient monitor.

The Patient Bedside Monitor
as a Data Management Terminal

Through a simple combination of function keys the data management window can be opened at a patient monitor. Neither the monitoring functionality nor the comprehensive alarm activation are lost or hindered because these actions have a higher priority. This can also be seen as a disadvantage, due to the fact that alarm activation at another patient monitor closes the data management window and the current alarm situation then appears on the screen. However, this is done for safety reasons and there is no compromise involved in such events.

As soon as new clinical findings have arrived, for instance results from the clinical laboratory, a message appears in small sized letters at the top of the patient monitor. This message is also supplemented by an acoustic signal. Upon opening the data management window at the patient monitor, the newest data is immediately shown, whereby pathological values are indicated by bold characters. Laboratory data are summarized individually in different groups. Groups for which the new lab data have arrived are also indicated optically by bold characters and can be brought up on the screen by command. The lab data is presented in cumulative form and in columns with the appropriate date and time. As soon as laboratory values are brought up within the data management window at the patient monitor, the lab values are considered validated and are stored in the database of the computer system.

A cumulative daily report can be printed at the central computer workstation which can be put together with the patient's record. Just as with the daily reports, a record of the vital-signs data can be printed within a user-defined time-interval which can also be included in the patient's documentation.

The multiprocessing operating system OS/2 enables the computer workstation to run other application software, like a word processor, simulations [5], expert systems or a spreadsheet program, without interrupting the automatic data acquisition from patient monitors.

All acquired parameters are stored centrally in the database of the server. This data can be called up and processed at each workstation on the network.

Through the open structure of the system, it is possible to place an application computer next to the bedside so that the entire set of trend curves and other wave forms can be stored at a bedside station. This would make a step-by-step extension of the system setup possible.

Experiences

The system described above has been on-line for the last six months as a clinical trial. The database is now comprised of approximately 400 patients.

In spite of a few performance faults, which are attributed to slow database access, the system has been stabile.

Bedside access to current laboratory data leads to faster decisions, thereby leading to an optimization of therapy [6,4]. Also, the on-line data acquisition of laboratory data has been a significant relief for the medical staff in the intensive care unit as well as for the laboratory personnel, because telephone contact or cooperative effort for collecting patient associated data is no longer necessary.

A study was conducted at the Klinik am Eichert to investigate the effects the system. During a 25 day period before and after the implementation of the system, the number of calls to the clinical laboratory and the amount of time required for each call was recorded.

Table 1. Effests of an on-line lab data transfer before and after implementation

	Before implementation	After implementation
Days of care	164	188
Number of calls	466	65
Calls/patients/day	2.84	0.34
Time/call (in minutes)	3.01	3.26
Time/year (in hours)	884.05[1]	114.63[1]
Cost/year (in DM)	35361.88	4585.08

[1] Time per year was multiplied by two (two people on the telephone)

At the same time the number of staff was also registered (see Table 1). Converted to a year (average occupancy is 8.5 patients/day), it was determined that the total time spent on the telephone was 884.05 hours per year. The resulting personnel costs came to be 35,361.88 DM per year, assuming the personnel cost to be 40 DM per hour. After implementing the system, the number of telephone calls to the laboratory were reduced to 65 (average time per call was 3.26 minutes) with 188 days of care (.34 calls/patient/day). After implementing the system, 114.3 hours per year would be necessary for obtaining laboratory values. The associated personnel costs would be 4,585.08 per year (see Figs. 2–4).

Through an open software structure and through the adherence to industry standards (operating system, SQL database, PC hardware), individual adaptation and system expansion according to departmental requirements are made possible. A comprehensive flow of data is achieved through the connection into a PC network. No redundant data is stored and by automatically securing data, the system prevents any loss of acquired information. At the same time, efficiency is optimized through the use of a PC network for administrative and statistical functions, as well as for expert systems. By establishing a link to the internal hospital information system, the transfer of patient demographics and documentation from various origins is possible. Through tying together an Acuity Scoring System, like detailed lists of items and their cost for each patient and quality assurance measures, the organizational structure and its needs can be described and the personnel requirements can thereby be determined or proven [5].

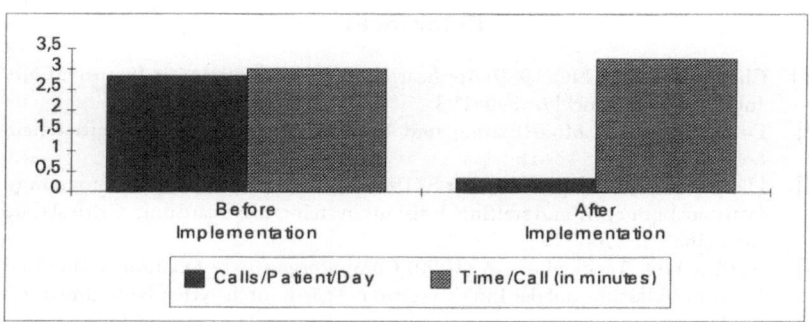

Fig. 2. Time and number of calls

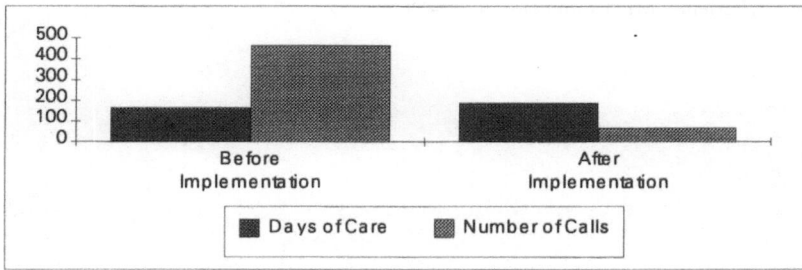

Fig. 3. Days of care and total number of calls

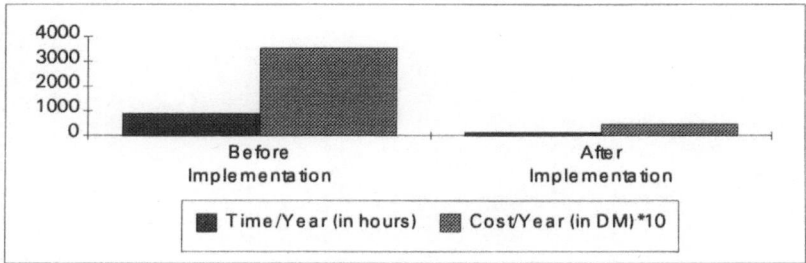

Fig. 4. Time and cost

References

[1]   Church JA, Gavin NC (1989) Applications of Microcomputers in Intensive Care. Intensive Care World 6: 190–193

[2]   Dzida W (1988) Modellierung und Bewertung von Benutzerschnittstellen. Software Kurier 1: 13–18

[3]   Hashimoto F, Bell S, Marshment S (1987) A computer simulation program to facilitate budgeting and staffing decisions in an intensive care unit. Critical Care Medicine 15: 256–259

[4]   Herden HN, Tecklenburg A (1990) Computergestützte Dokumentation und Leistungserfassung auf der Intensivstation. Anästh Intensivther Notfallmed 25: 79–82

[5]   Prentice JW, Kenny GNC (1986) Microcomputers in medical education. Medical Teacher 8: 9–17

[6]   Reed M, Gardner PP (1986) Computerized Management of Intensive Care Patients. MD Computing 3: 36–51

III. User Experiences

Problems and Experiences During the Installation of a PDMS

J. Wilding

Department of Inner Medicine IV, Intensive Care Unit,
University of Vienna, Austria

As we changed the location of our ICU to the newly built part of the hospital, we were confronted for the first time with the new PDMS for our ward. As we did not know that the computers were already installed at the new ICU, we were rather taken by surprise. At this time we neither had any information about this system, nor had we had the chance to see it before. Furthermore, the PDMS were not the only new machines in our ward. There were also new monitors, ventilators, and machines for hemodialysis. Therefore we had to spare a lot of time for lessons. Altogether this put an enormous stress on the care-personnel. And we had to give up our long-used and well-known written documentation.

In October we began to form a configuration-team together with the vendor. The leader of this team was a MD working for the computer-company. We did the configuration for all the ICUs on our floor. There are 3 medical ICUs and one acute-dialysis. We had separate configuration teams for the care personnel and for the physicians. Our team consisted of two nurses per station. In the following six months we met once a week for four hours, during the consecutive seven month we met twice monthly. Our work was to define all of the parameters of the system. This means a lot of flexibility for the system but also an enormous amount of work during implementation. People working with the system should know exactly what functions the system should provide. At this time we had no possibilities to make our work easier by comparison with other configurations. For instance, we had to arrange all of the menu-lists included in the system by ourselves. Each ward which plans to install a PDMS should know that the configuration of the system to the individual needs will take quite a while.

We started using the PDMS during our configuration work. Gradually we began to change from written documentation to the computer-system. Aware of the fear of data-loss, we did double documentation at the beginning: hand-written and computerized. This double-work means a lot of additional time needed for documentation. The first data which weren't saved on a written paper any more were the respirator-data. They are not transmitted automatically, but have to be entered manually into the system up to now.

The next step was the on-line take-over of the vital parameters from the patient monitor. This was the first real improvement since the start of the PDMS. In release E, which we are using now, the data have to be validated manually to be imported to the worksheet. Experiences show that this kind of validation has to be checked very carefully to ensure correct data. As an example, think of the registration of the CVD. With the new release F which will be installed this fall, we will have the choice between manual and automatic validation.

It took some time to overcome the doubts in doing the documentation only via PDMS. This was due to the fact that we had still had no training for the system. In addition it took some time for our colleagues to get used to the new system. It makes also a difference if the data are being entered into a computer-chart or into a hand-written chart. The following facts should be considered:

— It is not possible to enter free text in our system; for each category there is a list of presets wherefrom you can select only one for each cell of the worksheet. The problem that occurs is that you often would need more ways to describe a situation. For instance, think of a patient with a cataract and edema of the conjunctiva, and a defect of the cornea. If you have to describe the situation, which entry would you prefer: cataract, e.o.c. or corneal lesion? The nurses now have to decide which of this possibilities is the best. To make a decision as correctly possible is not very easy as you see. This problem did not occur during charting the data manually.

— In our ward there was an increase of the amount of data since the use of the PDMS. One of the underlying reasons is certainly the time-oriented scale of the system. All manipulations should be entered at the time of their performance. This leads to the situation that many of the nursing activities have to be entered repeatedly, even if this does not make much sense.

A great help in the assignment of conspicuous properties would be a graphical display of the human body. The written descriptions which have to be given instead also increase the amount of entered data. The short summary about the patient's day which was a valuable source of information at changing shifts was replaced by a confusing mass of data. This makes it difficult to divide the important from the unimportant facts.

Before medication and fluid balance were transferred to the computer system, the company trained 4 persons per ward in a 2 days training. Those nurses were trained as trainers themselves and had to train their colleagues in turn. These "trainers" had to do this during their routine activities, which was quite a burden for those nurses. When it became obvious that the training of 4 persons was not enough, the company added some more training lessons. Since most people can handle the system alike, training of new nurses is not a problem any more.

After the entire documentation had been transferred we had some problems with the unusual presentation of the patient data. Physicians as well as nurses were used to find all important data with one glance at the patient chart. It took some time to configure a "QUICK-LOOK" screen, which presents also the most important data on one screen. Nevertheless, it is still more time consuming to evaluate data from the PDMS than it was from our written documentation.

We got some program updates to cover most of the detected deficiencies. This had the advantage that the system got slowly but consistently adapted to our needs. For example, new parameters were added, unnecessary ones deleted. Still, until today the system's configuration is not optimized at all. It should be mentioned at this point that one of our main problems is in fact not a problem of the system-producer, but of our clinical information system. This CIS is not able to provide our PDMS with laboratory data. That means, that all laboratory data have to be managed by written documentation. This is the main reason why our documentation is still not transferred completely to the PDMS. The system speed is another difficulty we have to face. It still does not provide all information quickly enough. This causes problems with the change-over of shifts because it is unreasonable to wait more than a minute for a special information. Sometimes this leads to a lack of information.

Another problem which we did not expect was the big accumulation of printouts. As already stated, the same data is fed into the computer several times. The amount of paper used was enormous because all of these data were printed in hourly intervals, even when the majority of the printouts was rather useless. With a 2 or 4 hours printing interval the paper-flow is now reduced.

Finally it should be mentioned that it is possible to enter the same data in different parts of the chart. In this case it is not easy to find a common solution which satisfies all people. Moreover, the significance of the entered data is sometimes not precise enough to avoid different interpretations.

Conclusion

A good instruction of the care personnel helps to minimize the problems during installation. Following points should be mentioned:

- to see and compare different systems;
- to visit a ward where the system you want to purchase is already running fully in clinical use;
- to form a configuration-team prudently; it is recommendable that the same persons should be busy with that work the entire time, otherwise to avoid delays;
- an extensive training of all of the members of the ward, who have to work with the system later; this should not be done during routine work, but in special lessons.

Finally I want to say, that the work with the computer system motivates a lot of our colleagues very positively. At first we were all very critic at the unknown PDMS. The beginning was a time full of confrontation with a lot of deplores, because we were not used to work with the PDMS. The more the people became familiar with the system, the more it was accepted as a help in routine work. We hope development of our system is carried on so that a solution to our remainig problems may be found as soon as possible.

One Year Experience with a Unix-Based Clinical Information System (CIS) on an SICU

M. Imhoff

Chirurgische Klinik, Städtische Kliniken, Dortmund, Germany

Summary

The traditional handwritten documentation can by no means meet the continuously increasing demands in modern intensive care. In a clinical evaluation a unix-based CIS was tested on a major German surgical intensive care unit (SICU). After a short training period most of the documentation work could be done with the CIS. Time savings resulted from automatic calculations of intake/output summaries and hemodynamics, and from on-line data transfer from bedside devices. The 100% legibility of the computer documentation, its consistent structure and terminology, and its comprehensiveness provided for a major improvement in quality. Thus, in a first clinical testing in a German SICU the replacement of the handwritten record with a unix-based CIS was successful and advantageous.

Introduction

The necessity for bedside computing systems in hospitals, in general, and ICUs, in particular, has been repeatedly publicized in the last two decades [7, 23].

The patient record remains the principal instrument for ensuring the continuity of care. The numerous devices for intensive care monitoring and therapy combined with the steadily increasing acuity of our patients demand an improvement of integration and acquisition of patient data [10, 17].

Despite the increasing number of microprocessor controlled devices for monitoring and therapy most or all documentation is still done by hand. This discrepancy leads to a major reduction of information in a way that between 30 and 50% of all interventions and observations are not recorded, especially in emergency situations [4, 9, 13, 15, 20].

Therefore, the handwritten documentation has been expanded without really solving the underlying problems. In the Dortmund SICU the standard documentation comprises 12 to 16 pages A4 and additional documentation for therapeutic and diagnostic interventions.

Moreover, several studies and our own investigations show, that approximately 35% of the working hours of an ICU nurse are spent on documentation [12, 24].

In addition errors and mistakes in control and monitoring of therapy as well as forensic problems can no longer be ruled out [2, 8, 11, 18, 19].

Clinical Testing

Goals

The general goal of our investigation was to test the efficiency and adequacy of a unix-based CIS during daily routine of a major SICU in Germany.

In order to enable a comparison between the CIS and the old handwritten records some ICU beds were equipped with computers whereas others retained the old documentation. The clinical testing started on June 1, 1992. So far more than 1500 days of therapy have been documented with the CIS.

The following aspects were of particular interest:

- General technical testing in a clinical environment.
- Acceptance by the users.
- Reduction of handwritten documentation and replacement by the CIS.
- Changes in the quality of documentation and workload.

Architecture of the CIS

The CIS is based on a network of autonomous unix workstations, one for each bed. Bedside devices, such as monitors, ventilators, and IV devices, are connected locally via serial interfaces. All patient data is stored on the local harddisk at the bedside and simultaneously mirrored onto a second workstation within the network. This guarantees a 100% redundancy of data. An administrative data server is used for administration of the network (NIS) and CIS, and may serve as a communication hub with central data services, e.g. HIS, LIS.

The user interface is a mouse- and keyboard driven graphical user interface hased on X-windows, either in color or monochrome.

For testing the following hard- and software components were used:

- *Workstation:* Sun SPARCstation IPC/IPX (bedside), SPARCstation 2 (server, viewstation).
- *Patient Monitoring:* Siemens Sirecust 1280 with local interface to bedside workstation.
- *Network:* Ethernet, TCP/IP, NFS.
- *Operating System:* Sun OS 4.1.x, X11 Rel. 4 (Sun Open Windows).
- CIS: Siemens EMTEK System 2000 in German translation.

General Experience

The initial training with the new CIS was done with only a limited number of experienced critical care and respiratory nurses. After one to three days these nurses could work with the system on their own. Then this "core group" acted as tutors for other nurses and physicians. This step-wise approach allowed a smooth migration to the CIS even without special courses.

The following aspects of working with the CIS were most important for the users:

- On-line storage of all patient data allows an easy access and retrieval in case of a patient readmission or for retrospective analysis.
- Documentation is 100% legible. The system provides a consistent schema for data entry which allows easy retrieval of information.
- In emergency situations automatic data transfer allows to first deal with the patient and then to chart retrospectively after the problem is solved.
- As all workstations are integrated in a standard network, transparent and simultaneous data access from different workplaces is feasible.

— Both bedside devices and central data services can be interfaced.
   Among these patient monitor and ventilators at the bedside and the
   laboratory information system are the most importanl data sources.

The mouse as a digital pointing device was well accepted by all users.
An optical mouse seems advantageous for reasons of hygiene and
cleaning. With increased experience many users take advantage of a
simultaneous use of the keyboard and numerous function keys for
shortcuts.

Even users unfamiliar with keyboards describe a reduction of work
load and a significant enhancement in the quality of documentation.
The quality of the computer screens is essential in daily practice. A
resolution of 1 Megapixel on a 17" screen appears to be the minimum.
In direct comparison, monochrome display was preferred over color.

All functionality including database contents (parameters) and
layout are freely configurable. The configuration for the Dortmund
installation was done by trained medical personnel (one physician and
three nurses). Configuration by health care professionals, rather than by
computer specialists has proven efficient and successful in the current
installation and is strongly recommended by the author. This approach
allows swift reaction to new demands. Configuration itself, both for the
initial installation and for the running system, require profound
medical and clinical knowledge, whereas, the technicalities of the
conliguration process are straight-forward and easy to understand.

Quality and Efficiency of Documentation

Six weeks after the introduction of the system the handwritten documentation was discontinued for all sections that can be charted with the
CIS. This resulted in a reduction of the daily paperwork from 16 pages
to 2 pages, which actually is the remainder of the medical orders form.
These medical orders, in conjunction with the cardex will be replaced
by the CIS in the summer of 1993, so that a completely paperless
environment is available at the bedside.

Currently the following is charted with the CIS:

— *Vital Signs:* All vital signs are charted with the CIS. Most parameters are transferred on-line from the patient monitor. In addition
   comprehensive item list for e.g. arrhythmia are available. Numer-

ous calculations (hemodynamics, oxygen transport) are done automatically.

- *Ventilation:* All ventilation parameters are charted in a dedicated ventilation flowsheet.
- *Neurological assessment:* The neurological status is documented with the help of item for up to 63 parameters. A precise and comprehensive assessment and the calculation of neurological scores is feasible even for the inexperienced user without additional workload.
- *Intake/Output:* The complete charting of fluid intake and output (I&O) is done with the CIS. Even extended I&O chart can be displayed in a comprehensible way, as there are no limitations in charting space. I&O summaries are available for freely configured intervals as well as for totals, running totals and subgroups. In addition electrolyte and nutritional calculations are integrated in I&O. Calculation errors are eliminated and up to 45 minutes can be saved per day per patient. IV device interfaces are a solved technical issue. Nevertheless, interfacing IV devices has to be seen critically because so far automatic identification of drugs and infusions is not available in any IV devices presently marketed.
- *Lab tests:* All lab test results are directly transferred from the LIS via an HL-7 link, if available in the respective hospital.
- *Notes:* Notes can be entered as free text or from lists of text blocks, both in a dedicated notes section and from within each individual data cell. Notes are structured and can be retrieved and searched following topics and subtopics and in chronological order.
- *Nursing procedure charting:* The documentation of nursing, care and patient observation is done in a dedicated tabular flowsheet and with additional notes. At the moment the adaption of the US care plans integrated in the CIS to German standards is under investigation.
- *Cost calculations:* In a first step toward an automatic accounting system, on-line cost calculations for drugs and infusions were integrated in the I&O section. This allows accurate assessment of the effective medication costs for every individual patient.

Despite an initial scepticism the parallel use of a paperless documentation (CIS) at the bedside, and the conventional documentation and archiving of diagnostic and administrative data did not cause any problems.

Communication with other units and departments within and outside the hospital is still based on paper records. Upon transfer or discharge of a patient, the complete electronic chart is printed. In this case the printout takes the medico-legal position of the old handwritten record. Due to the enhanced comprehensiveness of the CIS and the overall acuity of the patients the average record fills between 12 and 20 pages per day and patient. Thus, in contrast to computerized imaging systems (e.g. PACS), saving in archiving volume cannot be expected at the moment.

Discussion

More than one year of clinical evaluation showed that a unix-based CIS can replace the traditional handwritten record on a German SICU and provide a major improvement in daily practice. These results correspond to investigations in the US.

In US ICUs time savings of 30 to 90 minutes per shift per nurse could be observed [6, 16, 21, 22].

Quality of documentation is difficult to measure. Two independent studies have found a reduction in medication errors of between 30 and 40% [5, 22]. In our evaluation a significant improvement in quality was achieved by standardized and precise item and menu lists, as well as by the extensive options to describe and monitor the current status of the patient.

The importance of interfacing with central data services, such as LIS and HIS, is emphasized by Lappa [14]. Investigations by Bradshaw et al. [3] support this, as 42% of all central data result from lab test.

The connection with central data services needs a logistic setting that has to be provided by the respective hospital. The problem of interfaces to bedside devices can, in the long run, only be solved by a general standardization at reasonable cost. This would need a commitment by all vendors.

Besides better patient care through improved quality and efficiency of documentation emphasis has to be put on the forensic aspects of the patient record. The recent problems, especially those of liabilities, can be addressed much better with professional CIS [1, 18].

References

[1] Barrett JJ, Saltz VW (1991) Potential liability for defective expert systems. Annual International Conference of the IEEE Engineering in Medicine and Biology Society 13: 1347–1348

[2] BGH vom 23. 11. 1982 – MedR 1982, S. 62

[3] Bradshaw KE, Gardner RM, Clemmer TP, et al (1984) Physician decision-making – Evaluation of data used in a computerized ICU. Int J Clin Monit Comput 1: 81–9110

[4] Brimm JE (1987) Computers in critical care. Crit Care Nurs 9: 53–63

[5] Cerne F (1989) Study finds bedside terminals prove their worth. Hospitals 63: 729

[6] Donovan W, Corrales S (1991) The book on bedside computing. Inside Healthcare Computing, Long Beach, CA

[7] Dzida W (1988) Modellierung und Bewertung von Benutzerschnittstellen. Software Kurier 1: 13–28

[8] Furst E (1989) Computerizing the intensive care unit: Current status and future directions. J Cardiovasc Nurs 4: 68–78

[9] Gardner RM (1987) Computer technology and its application to cardiovascular nursing. J Cardiovasc Nurs 1: 69–71

[10] Gardner RM, Sittig DF, Budd MC (1989) The computer in the ICU: Match or mismatch? In: Textbook of Critical Care Medicine, 2nd edn. WB Saunders, Philadelphia

[11] Gardner RM, Shabot MM (990) Computerized ICU data management: pitfalls and promises. Int J Clin Monit Comput 7: 99–105

[12] Imhoff M (1991) Datenerfassung in der Patientenüberwachung – Problemstellung und Lösungsmöglichkeiten. Anaesthesist 40 [Suppl 2]: 132

[13] Imhoff M (1992) Acquisition of ICU data: concepts and demands. Int J Clin Monit Comput 9: 229–237

[14] Lappa K (1989) Inpatient bedside system enters the computer age. Hospitals 63: 769

[15] Larsen JL, Jenkins JM (1987) Computerized arrhythmia monitoring. J Cardiovasc Nurs 1: 58–66

[16] Leyerle BJ, LoBue M, Shabot M (1990) Integrated computerized databases for medical data management beyond the bedside. Int J Clin Monit Comput 7: 83–89

[17] McDonald CJ, Tierney WM (1988) Computer-stored medical records: Their future role in medical practice. JAMA 259: 3433–3440

[18] Narr H (1989) Ärzliches Berufsrecht. Band 2. 11. Ergänzung. Deutscher Ärzteverlag, Köln. S. 5757

[19] OLG Karlsruhe v. 21. 07. 1982 – MedR 1983, S. 147

[20] Opderbecke u. Weißauer – MedR 1984, S. 211

[21] Shabott MM, LoBue M, Leyerle BJ, Dubin SB (1990) Decision support alerts for clinical laboratory and blood gas data. In J Clin Monit Comput 7: 27–31

[22] Shelton CR (1989) Bedside Computers Hospital Friendly? New Jersey Healthcare 3–6

[23] Villalobos J, Manzano J, Blazquez M, Bolanos J, Lubillo S (1986) Computerized system in intensive care medicine. Med Inform 11: 269–275

[24] Wendt M, Booke M, Hörauf K (1991) Datenflut in der Patientenüberwachung – Konzepte zur Optimierung des Datenmanagements. Anaesthesist 40 [Suppl 2]: 133

User Experiences with Patient-Data-Management-Systems (PDMS) at Four International Sites

H. Andel and G. Schak

Department of Anaesthesia and General Intensive Care,
University of Vienna, Austria

Introduction

Four different clinical departments (University Hospital Antwerpen, Belgium, University Hospital Lund, Sweden, Cedars Sinai, L.A., USA, LAC University Hospital, L.A., USA), using three different PDMS (Marquette-PDMS/Clinicomp, CareVue 9000/Hewlett Packard, Siemens-PDMS/Emtek) were visited in December 1992.

University Hospital Antwerpen, Belgium

Department:	Internal ICU (Prof. Leo Bossaert)
	Heart surgery ICU, Neonatal ICU
Date:	07. 12. 1992
Beds:	25
PDMS:	Marquette-PDMS / Clinicomp (2 SUN mainframes with X-terminals, UNIX Operating system, StarLAN network), monochrome display.
Interfaces:	Patient monitor Marquette, HIS (central lab, local lab, demographic data), ventilator (as of March 1993)

Observations

The system has been installed for one and a half years, but has only been in operation since November 18th, 1992. The users are satisfied with certain limitations. Despite massive problems in the implementation phase the system has now been accepted.

Data entering is done solely via keyboard with the help of the function keys. As of the end of December 1992 some terminals will be equipped with a trackball on a trial basis. Data entering is time consuming and complicated, whereby even the trainer, despite system experience, often pressed the wrong function key. The PDMS is constantly connected via modem with the headquarters of the company in San Diego, California. Revisions in configuration are incorporated in the program, and when possible, are realized by a team of technicians in California within 24 hours.

User training followed the "Train-the-Trainer"-principle over a period of ten days.

During clinical visits PDMS is partially used, whereby lab results and the extensive graphic features support the physicians decision. PDMS is only partially used by the nursing staff. Utilization is restricted, at change of shift, to laboratory data. Nursing particulars are still done by hand.

A scientific evaluation of patient data is at present not in practise. With appropriate training, a systems engineer (technician), should be able to perform an evaluation.

The archiving of patient data is in the form of printouts and hand written notes; digital immediately on an optical disc, as well as shadowing via modem in San Diego, California.

The maintenance costs account for 7-8 percent of the procurement cost, whereby the modem alone accounts for AS 500.000 per year.

The reduction in paper work for personnel is approximated at 50 percent.

University Hospital Lund, Sweden

Department:	Anaesthesia ICU (Dr. Anders Larssen), Recovery room
Date:	08. 12. 1992
Beds:	9 + 3 recovery beds
PDMS:	HP CareVue 9000/ Hewlett Packard (Cluster of bedside discless workstations with a fileserver pair, UNIX Operating system, StarLAN), colour display.
Interfaces:	Patient monitor HP Merlin, central lab, local lab, ventilator (as of April 1993)

Observations

The system has been in operation since May 1991. A generally good acceptance by users is reported.

Data entering is done via keyboard with the connected trackball. A major part of data entering can be done via trackball alone.

The display design is structured in graphics and lines, facilitating a flexible display design.

The PDMS, for the practised user, can be easily adapted with the help of configuration tools with graphic features to accomodate clinical necessities. Formulas for calculations can be added or edited. The system is serviced by two HP employees and is connected via modem to the local response centre of the producer.

User training followed the "Train-the-Trainer"-principle over a period of two days.

PDMS is not used during clinical visits, but the visits are assisted by printouts.

Printouts are also used at the change of shifts by the nursing staff, although nursing particulars are still done by hand.

A scientific evaluation of patient data is at present not practised. An extraction via ASCII-format followed by additional processing using the database PARADOX is planned for the first quarter of 1993.

At present manual records as well as printouts of the PDMS are filed. Computer assisted archiving is not in use.

As yet there has been no savings using the PDMS. Time saving for nursing personnel is approximated at 20 percent.

University Hospital Cedars Sinai, Los Angeles, USA

Department: General surgery ICU, liver transplantation ICU
               (Prof. M. Shabot, Beverly J. Leyerle, Mark LoBue)
Date: 09. 12. 1992
Beds: 16
PDMS: HP CareVue 9000 / Hewlett Packard (Cluster of bed-
               side discless workstations with a fileserver-pair, UNIX
               Operating system, StarLAN), colour display.
Interfaces: Patient monitor HP Merlin, central lab, Puritan Ben-
               net ventilator, self-developed interface drivers using
               UNIX.

Observations

The system has been in operation since 1990. An exceptionally good acceptance by users is reported.

Data entering is done via keyboard with the connected trackball.

The PDMS, for the practised user, can be easily adapted with the help of configuration tools with graphic features to accomodate clinical necessities. This task is accomplished by three hospital employees (Director Prof. Shabot, nursing manager, technician).

At present the system is being serviced by an internal technician and an employee of the producer Hewlett Packard, whereby close contact is upheld with the development department of the producer (Beta-Site). Additionally a modem connection with the local response centre of HP exists.

Independent software applications were developed. This enables a direct connection to the HP CareVue 9000 system.

The internal applications consist of a collation of fluid balances as well as the laboratory parameter in an especially clear presentation together with the corresponding printout.

Clinical visits are largely PDMS supported. Special printouts are also produced via the internal UNIX-applications. At change of shifts HP CareVue 9000 as well as internal applications printouts are used.

PDMS data is automatically incorporated into the UNIX database for scientific evaluation. At present, data of some 12,000 patients are available for evaluation. Sundry scores are calculated with the internal applications (an internal score consisting of 125 parameters has been developed). Due to legal aspects hand-signed printouts of the PDMS and the internal applications are filed.

Support of the system is done by a technician employed by the hospital. In case of a problem, primarily the system manager of the hospital (Prof. Shabot, nursing manager, technician) is available around the clock.

Functions in the sense of a Decision Review System are only marginally available (in the case of a major reduction in the haemoglobin level within a defined period of time the display issues a warning).

With the aid of internal system specialists an optimum adaptation of the system to the particular units' needs has been achieved. The further development in the sense of a Decision Review System has only been possible with the efforts of these system specialists. Unforeseen operating costs have so far not occurred, though the system specialists' salary is paid by the hospital.

Time saving for nursing personnel is approximated at 50 percent.

University Hospital Southern California, Los Angeles, USA

Department:	2 Surgery ICU (Focus: Traumatology)
Date:	10. 12. 1992
Beds:	20
PDMS:	Emtek / Motorola (SUN-Sparcstations with a central fileserver), monochrome display
Interfaces:	Patient monitor HP Merlin, central lab, local lab, Siemens Servo 900 ventilator

Observations

The system has been in operation since 1991. The users are satisfied without exception.

Data entering is done via keyboard and function keys, as well as an optical mouse. Graphics or lines are optional. Display can be suited to each individual patient. The system, with the aid of an Emtek engineer, is constantly adaptable to clinical needs. At present only the engineer is able to modify the configuration.

Training is supplied by a nurse of the institution with computer experience.

The physician and nurse clinical visits utilize fully the PDMS system.

With the aid of simple word processing, nursing notes can be registered, whereby the remarks made can be arranged independently.

For the next software version the implementation of a Decision Research Workstation is planned.

An Emtek engineer supports the incumbent researcher. A direct SQL-tool is available, but a more user-friendly application is planned.

Archiving is done regularly on magnetic data tape, although, due to legal reasons, printouts of patient data is also filed.

An Emtek engineer is available for around the clock maintenance. The engineer is home-based, and equipped with a modem, in order to tackle problems promptly.

The operation costs amount to approx. 300,000 AS per month (incl. Emtek engineer). Time saving for the nursing staff is approximated at 50 percent.

Conclusion

At all sites the users were pleased working with a PDMS. Each department uses paper-based patient documentation additionally. An interface to the Hospital Information System is realized in all cases. At all sites the clinical consultation was at least supported by the PDMS. Time savings when using PDMS are reported to be 20–50 percent. The most impressive visit was at the Cedars Sinai Hospital. At this site with a HP CareVue 9000, a technician was able to develop his own application which runs on the same hardware, adding archiving and scientific research functions to the application.

As this example shows the utilization of hospital technicians, interested in PDMS development, allows the adaptation on specific clinical demands.

Information System for ICU.
The Finnish Hospitals' Consortium

A. Heikelä and A. Nyberg

Clinisoft Ltd, Kuopio, Finland

There are only few data management systems in daily use in Europe. The systems have usually been developed for one unit. Therefore the functional and data requirements have been limited. In the AIM-Inform project (1989-1990) the objective was to bring together a larger group of clinicians and computer scientists. The project resulted in firm overall specifications for a data management system. The Finnish Technical Research Centre as well as Helsinki and Kuopio University Central Hospitals participated in that project.

There was a clear need to specify the users' requirements so exactly and widely that a next generation data management system could be designed. The basis for this aim was to utilise existing knowledge and to get a wide clinical expertise through consortium approach.

In 1991–92 eleven Finnish hospitals established a consortium. There were 4 university hospitals and 7 central hospitals. The project group included also the Medical Engineering Laboratory of Finnish Technical Research Centre and the software house Clinisoft.

Aim of the Project

The aim of the project was to specify users' functional and data requirements for an information system. The target environment was an adult mixed surgical-medical ICU, but special needs of pediatric or specialized units were also included in the specifications.

The scope of the specifications was both patient and unit management. The former includes e.g. nursing activities, medication, fluid and respiratory therapy as well as patient administration. The latter e.g. resource management, cost accounting, quality assurance and inventory.

The other aim was to standardise the documentation of care, which then enables data exchange, nation-wide follow-up studies and the comparison of units. Special attention was paid on long-term unit management.

Overall Requirements for the System

The consortium set requirements for the planned system. The system should be very flexible, so that without reprogramming it could be adapted into different clinical units. It should be interfaced with medical devices and other hospital information systems. The user should be able to configure the functions and reports of the system. The system should be open for future decision support systems. Finally, the system should be economically feasible – to keep the requirements realistic.

Project Organisation

The project was controlled by a managing board, which had representatives from all participating hospitals and Finnish Hospitals League. The expert group was set up by managing board and authorised to advise and control the project group. In expert group there were representatives of nurses, physicians, computer experts and engineers.

Each hospital had a working group. In addition to clinicians there were technical experts.

Working Method

The project group prepared all draft specifications with the expert group. Thereafter all hospitals were visited three times for discussions. Finally, the expert group accepted the revised specifications. During the third visit a prototype was used to illustrate the specifications.

Specifications

Intensive care functions and their data contents were first described in textual form. With these we agreed upon the terminology and the functions to be included in the planned system. The system was then outlined with user requirements.

System modelling included formal descriptions of the functions and data. Thereafter the models depicting user-system dialogues were exemplified with a graphic design tool. Finally the specifications were illustrated in more details by prototyping the system.

The medical device and hospital information system environments were examined and the interfacing requirements with them were defined. The medico-legal standards as well as the information technological requirements were specified.

In addition to specifications the user group agreed upon the use of e.g. certain scoring systems and classifications. This kind of a standardisation will make it possible to exchange data between units, compare units and carry out nation-wide studies.

Conclusions

A project approach has several benefits for the hospitals. During the project the hospitals can discuss with experts of possibilities of information technology in intensive care. The users are also better aware about their needs and can demand them.

Working in a group decreases also the workload and costs of one hospital.

Only a wide clinical support can provide a system with full clinical functionality.

Final Note

In spring 1993 the Finnish consortium decided to choose Clinisoft system as the standard of patient data management system for intensive care in Finland.

Commercial Aspects in the Acquisition of Patient Data Management Systems

W. Perkmann

Hewlett Packard Medical Systems Group, Vienna, Austria

The increasing importance of information technology in the area of health care, especially hospitals, will certainly present a decisive key factor in the future success of such institutions. The development of feasible and functioning information systems in the medical profession is in constant evolution and finds resonance in the utilization thereof in hospitals. More and more feasible and functioning information systems are being developed for the medical market and are being released for use in hospitals.

Hospital managers need to face this challenge in order to take adequate decisions and to develop strategies to utilize information systems effectively in the interest of patients and employees.

Necessity, user-friendliness, economic viability, security, state-of-the-art and compatibility of system integration are important factors in the evaluation, planning and realization of PDM systems.

The successful investment and introduction of PDM systems in the intensive-care unit and in the operating theatre requires a comprehensive systems analysis with setting on objective, analysis of status quo, development of a target situation as well as the achievement of a complex evaluation method in the problem-solving process. This is a prerequisite for precise allotment, detailled planning and economic viability in the implementation of the project.

The better a PDM system can be integrated into an existing Hospital Clinical Information System, the more rational it is. Thus, planning and system analysis are interdependent and should be examined as a whole. The decision, whether to invest or not, should not be based on the possible nonprofitability of a relatively small area, but on the profitability of the entire, as a cost utilization relationship is difficult to determine on such a small scale.

Both buyer and producer should not only concentrate on the technical and operational evaluation of the system but should also agree on economic aspects and possible subjective trends involved. This will result in the successs of the product on market-place.

Although the market is technical oriented, evaluation of a PDM system is ultimately closely related to the public, and thus economic acceptance thereof. Thus, a market-orientated evalutation of a PDM system is closely related to methods of acceptance research. Methods frequently used comprise system analysis, market analysis, user questionnaires and also subjective evaluation techniques.

Conclusion

The selection of a PDM system first of all depends on the required application and the functionalities.

It depends on the system architecture, which enables certain functions and thus influences the decision to buy.

And last but not least, it depends on the operational management and operation costs both of which are key parameters in the decision to invest.

IV. Clinical Applications

Clinical Application of Patient Data Management Systems (PDMS): Computer-Assisted Weaning from Artificial Ventilation (KBWEAN)

M. Hiesmayr, J. Gamper, T. Neugebauer, P. Mares,
K. P. Adlassnig, and W. Haider

Department of Cardiothoracic Anaesthesia and Intensive Care Medicine,
Research Institute for Intensive Care Medicine,
Department of Medical Informatics, University of Vienna, Austria

Introduction

Since the early sixties expert systems for weaning of patients from artificial ventilation have been designed. The general approach as well as the chosen endpoints varied widely [1–10]. Since clinical results have been published by only few groups [10, 8], the practical use of these systems appears to be very limited. Recently published data on specific parts of the weaning process are encouraging [11–14]. They reported shorter weaning periods, a diminished number of blood gases [11, 8] or a greater percent of ventilation in the zone of confort [10].

Weaning remains a central point of interest for many intensivists because of two major problems. On the one hand an unsuccessful early weaning trial may precipitate respiratory muscle fatigue and the formation of atelectasis whereas on the other hand a delayed weaning increases the risk of nosocomial infection or may waste the limited capacity of many intensive care units. Usually weaning is done in a stepwise approach.

The goal of an improved weaning approach would be to make the transition from total dependency (controlled ventilation) to total independency (extubation) as smooth and short as possible.

Since the implementation of a PDMS in our unit and the integration of continously available signals from pulseoximetry (S_pO_2) and Capnometry (E_t CO_2) in the monitoring concept a specific expert system (KBWEAN) is developed to achieve these goals. This combination of a PDMS with an expert system should enlarge the PDMS from a documenting and trending device, what we consider to be a passive behaviour to a more active one as a clinical tool.

The aim of this study is the description of the system together with the underlying weaning concept and the presentation of our preliminary results in patients.

PDMS and Monitoring Setup

- The Monitoring setup includes 3 devices for vital signs, respiratory and ventilatory assessment:
  - Monitor: Mennen Horizon: Heartrate, blood pressures, cardiac output, body temperature, respiratory rate (RespRate)
  - Oximeter Capnometer Datex Oscar: Pulsoximetry (S_pO_2), endtidal CO_2 (E_tCO_2), respiratory rate (RespR)
  - Ventilator Dräger Evita (Software 9): inspired oxygen fraction (FiO_2), airway pressures (PEAK, PEEP), tidal volume, minute volume.
- These 3 devices are connected to an IBM PC (Mod. 70 386) via a multiserial card. All PC's are connected to a server via an IBM Token Ring Network.
- Software requirements: Deskview (2.4), Atlantis 1.42 (Hospitronics-Dräger), Novell Netware (3.11), KBWEAN (Medical Informatics Vienna).

Structure of the Knowledge-Based Expert System (KBWEAN)

The PDMS stores the sampled data in a file on the local disk as well as on the PDMS fileserver. KBWEAN reads this file and performs an analysis of the data at any time when a new record is appended to the file. KBWEAN runs with the local datafile or may analyze any file stored on the fileserver.

In a first step intervals that represent qualitative knowledge according to predefined endpoints have been formulated for all used parameters. These intervals are defined as normal, high, low, very high, very low and invalid data.

In the next step these categorised data are combined in IF...THEN rules with comparative (<, <=, =, >=, >, in interval), logical (and, or, not) and arithmetic (+, −, *, /) operators.

Example 1:

Rule OXYGENATION_2
if   not   [S_pO_2 normal or very low]
        and   [FiO_2 normal]
        and   [PEEP normal or low]
then
"LowPress +2 & HighPress +2"

A time oriented operator (ago(parameter,time)) allows a tracking of trends and of the effects of real not only proposed changes in therapy.

Example 2:

Rule TIME_5
if   [AGO ($EtCO_2$,30) − $EtCO_2$ >= 5
        and   [$EtCO_2$ high]
then
"Ventilation is improving −> no change!!"

Currently an improved and more robust trending operator is developed that works by describing and analysing states.

If a rule is true then the conclusion is displayed on the screen together with the dataset that was analysed. For further information a menu allows an extensive view of each rule in the rule file. The conclusions are in general a proposal of changes on the ventilator settings for the attending physician or the responsible nurse. A certain number of rules is used for "smart alarming". The consequences taken by the staff can be entered into a data screen, when a change is done. This information will also be available to the Expert System.

The actual rule set is designed for the ventilatory management with the BIPAP mode (Dräger Evita) since this mode allows a very smooth and gradual change from controlled to spontaneous breathing. In this pressure controlled mode 5 different parameters can be set [FiO_2, upper

(HighPress) and lower (LowPress) pressure level as well as the duration of each pressure level (HighTime, LowTime)]. These parameters are used in the conclusions according to the experiences from a "manual" weaning study in postoperative cardiac patients (n = 10), where the weaning steps were done every other hour. These patients were our actual study group. The proposed changes from KBWEAN will be compared to the actual changes done by the attending physician.

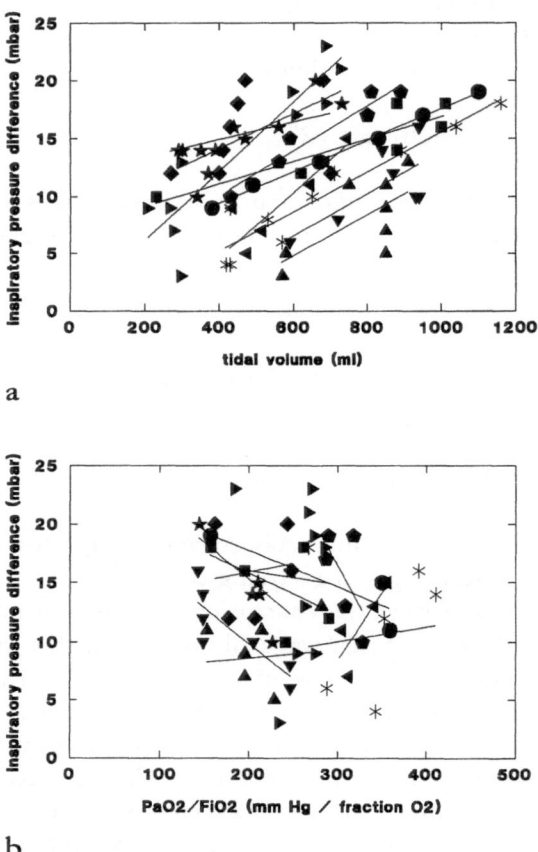

Fig. 1. Lung function during weaning: a Relationship of the difference HighPress-LowPress to tidal volume during weaning with the BIPAP mode (see text) with the individual regression lines for each patient (n = 10). b Relationship of the Oxygenation index to the difference HighPress-Lowpress

When the system is used in a postoperative patient the first settings represent those that were used in the operation theater just before the transport to the Intensive Care Unit. This corresponds usually to HighPress = 22–26 mbar for 2 seconds, LowPress = 6 mbar for 4 seconds and an FiO_2 of 60%. The resulting tidal volume is 8–10 ml/kg.

The weaning concept for oxygenation is that at first FiO_2 should be reduced as fast as possible to a level below 45% [15], in order to avoid atelectasis formation and have very low difference from ventilator FiO_2 to room air before extubation. When oxygenation deteriorates the first step would an increase in both pressure levels by an amount (2–4 mbar) that is guided by the previous settings and the amount of hypoxia. In traditional ventilatory treatment this corresponds to a change in PEEP. In a further step before FiO_2 is increased above 60% a decrease in expiratory time to achieve some air trapping in diseased lung areas is considered [16]. The effectiveness of oxygenation is based on pulsoximetry (S_pO_2) and the measured lower pressure level (PEEP) and FiO_2.

The weaning concept for ventilation is at first that the ventilatory peak pressures (upper level) should be as low as possible for adequate CO_2 elimination and secondly that the tidalvolume given by the ventilator should not exceed 12 ml/kg BW and is ideally about 8 ml/kg BW. Whenever the measured values are in the ideal zone, a reduction of upper level pressure by 2 mbar is done. This change corresponds to a change in tidal volume of 1 ml/kg as shown in Fig.1a by the individual regression lines of the change in tidal volume when HighPress is progressively decreased during the weaning process. Interestingly during this continuous decrease in ventilatory pressure no deterioration in the Oxygenation index (PaO_2/FiO_2) occurred (Fig. 1 b). The effectiveness of ventilation is judged by E_tCO_2, tidal volume, respiratory rate and minute ventilation as well as the measured inspiratory pressures (PEAK).

On the screen in a Deskview Window the actual values and proposed actions are shown and it is also possible to scroll the history back.

In addition to the screen display all measured data, activated rules and all actions that were documented by the staff are sampled in a database file with a dbase structure that allows easy post processing.

Two routine weaning courses and the online proposals of the system are shown in Fig. 2.

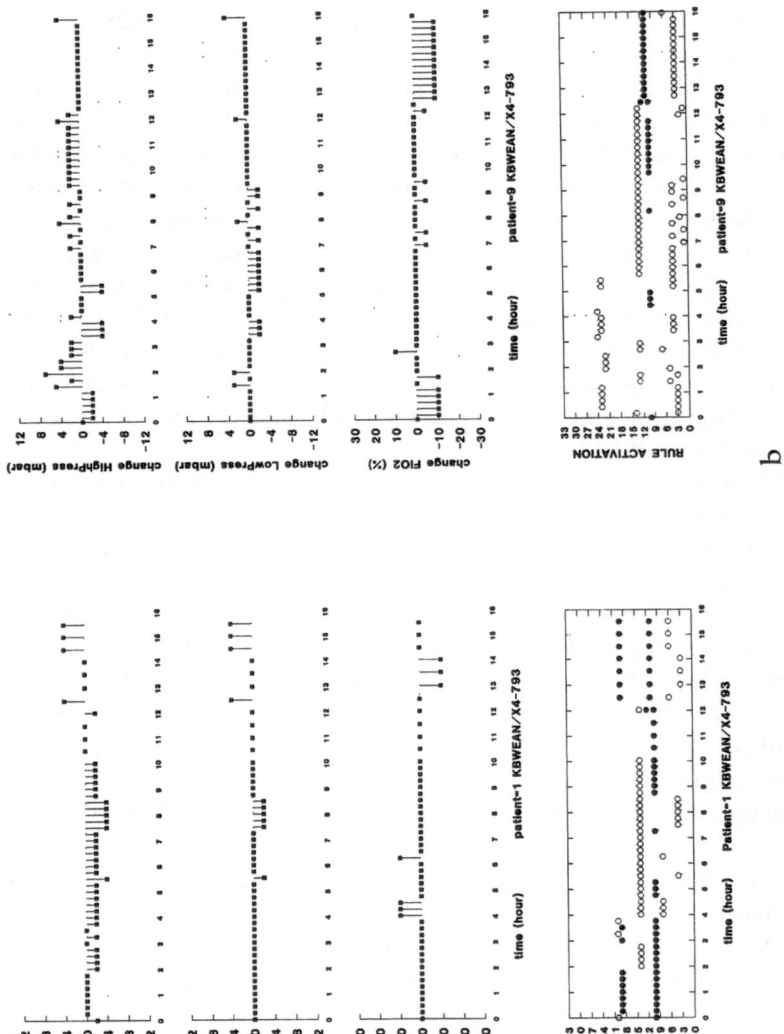

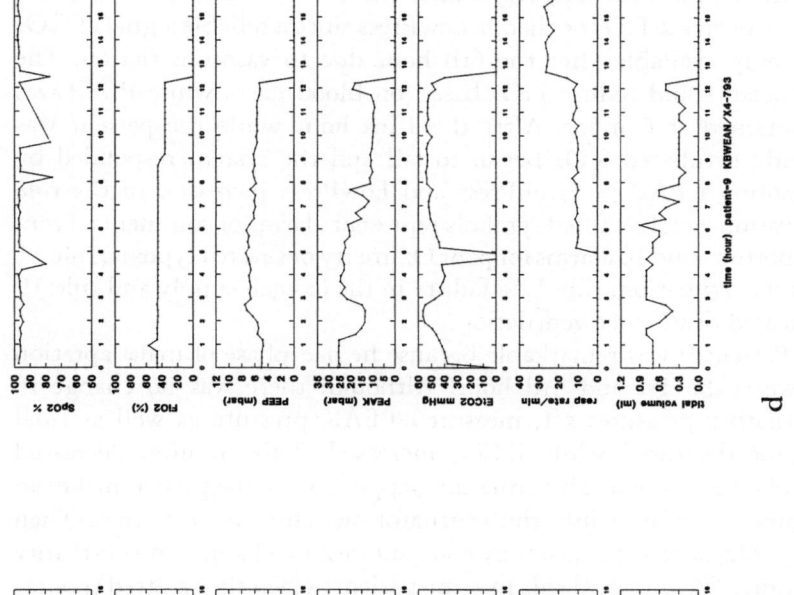

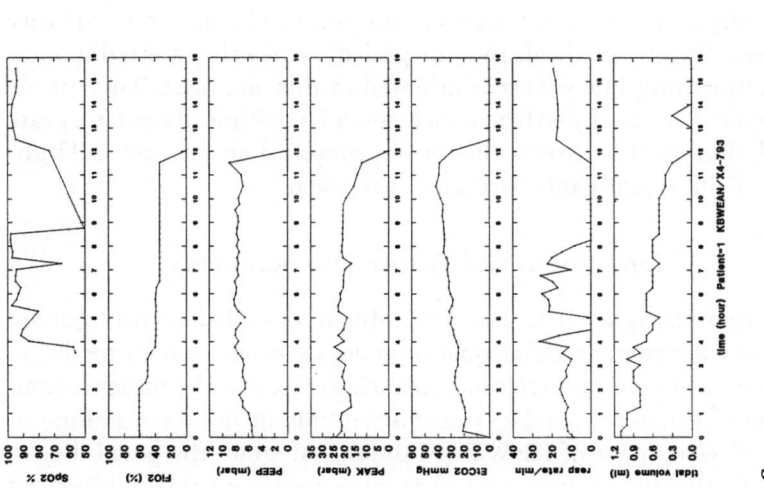

Fig. 2. KBWEAN advices during weaning in Patient 1 and 9. For details and interpretation see text

Patient 1 had an uncomplicated weaning course and was extubated after 11.5 hours. At first KBWEAN proposed very early (2nd hour) a HighPress reduction that has also been done by the attending physician. During this period tidal volume decreased progressively, while respiratory rate rose to 25 resp/min at the 4th hour. The system was not able to decrease FiO_2 or change LowPress since a reliable signal of S_pO_2 was only available after the 6th hour due to vasoconstriction. The physician could reduce FiO_2 based on blood gases while PEEP was maintained at 6 mbar. After the 14th hour while the patient was already extubated S_pO_2 began to fall and the system responded by proposing CPAP (= HighPress and LowPress increase). In the rule activation panel all filled symbols represent alarms or comments. From the bottom rule 10 alarms for poor Oximetry or severe Hypoxia, rule 11 detects extubation, rule 12 a failure in the oxygen supply and rule 19 increased dead space ventilation.

Patient 9 was remarkable because he had phase of maladaptation between the 1st and 3rd hour. Although there was no change in ventilatory pressures set, measured PEAK pressure as well as tidal volume decreased while E_tCO_2 increased. This signifies decreased alveolar ventilation. This situation happens when the patient makes an inspiratory effort while the ventilator switches to expiration. Then lung volume is kept relatively constant despite changes in ventilatory pressure. We observed this in some patients when they started spontaneous breathing but were not oriented at that moment. This can be overcome in 3 ways by either an increase in HighPress, Respiratory rate or sedation. In this patient the system proposed an increase in HighPress, while actually more sedation was given.

Limitations and Future Developments

These two examples show 2 major problems of such an expert system. First such a system needs adequate signals, that may be missing due to physiological (vasoconstriction, shivering), technical problems (motion) or less than perfect data transmitted from devices (ventilators). A future development of KBWEAN should integrate the possibility to ask for further information or an alternative measurement as a blood gas analysis for example. Secondly all points of the interaction between man and ventilator [17–19] in various modes of supported ventilation have still to be clarified. One of the problems is the clear detection of the onset of spontaneous breathing when the signals are noisy and the ventilatory mode is pressure driven with a very narrow triggering window.

Conclusion

- The extension of our PDMS with an expert system KBWEAN has been technically solved.
- This integrated approach allowed the exclusive use of continuously available variable for the weaning process. But the problem of incomplete or invalid data has to be solved.
- The use of continously available variables allows a much faster and smoother adptation to the patients needs than the traditional approach with intermittent blood gases.
- A larger study has to be done to identify the gaps in the rules and to find a minimal/optimal set.
- In the future an adaptation of the system to each individual patient (group of patients/diseases) could be necessary.

Literatur

[1] Fagan LM, Kunz JC, Feigenbaum EA, Osborn JJ (1984) Extensions to the rule-based formalism for a monitoring task (VM) in rule-based expert systems (Buchanan BG, Shortliffe EH, eds.). Addison-Wesley, Reading

[2] Miller PL (1985) Goal-directed critiquing by computer ventilator management. Computers and Biomedical Research 18: 422–438

[3] Hernandez-Sande C, Moret-Bonillo V, Alonso-Betanzos A (1989) ESTER: An expert system for management of respiratory weaning therapy. IEEE Transactions on Biomedical Engineering 36: 559–564

[4] Rudowski R, Frostell C, Gill H (1989) A knowledge-based support system for mechanical ventilation of the lungs. The KUSIVAR concept and prototype. Computer Methods and Programs in Biomedicine 30: 59–70

[5] Sittig DF, Gardner RM, Pace NL, Morris AH, Beck E (1989) Computerized management of patient care in a complex, controlled clinical trial in the intensive care unit. Computer Methods and Programs in Biomedicine 30: 77–84

[6] Shahsavar N, Frostell C, Gill H, Ludwigs U, Matell G, Wigertz O (1989) Knowledge base design for decision support in respirator therapy. Int J of Clin Monit and Comput 6: 223–231

[7] Tong DA (1991) Weaning patients from mechanical ventilation. A knowledge-based system approach. Computer Methods and Programs in Biomedicine 35: 267–278

[8] Strickland JH, Hasson JH (1991) A computer-controlled ventilator weaning system. Chest 100: 1096–1099

[9] Gärtner K (1992) Interaktive Beatmungsoptimierung mit dem Beratungs-system IBEUS. Biometrie und Informatik in Medizin und Biologie 23: 236–241

[10] Dojat M, Brochard L, Lemaire F, Harf A (1992) A knowledge-based system for assisted ventilation of patients in intensive care units. Int J of Clin Monit and Comput 9: 251–257

[11] Niehoff J, DelGuercio C, LaMorte W, Hughes-Grasberger SL, Heard S, Dennis R, Yeston N (1988) Efficacy of pulse oximetry and capnometry in postoperative weaning. Crit Care Med 16: 701–705

[12] Yang KL, Tobin MJ (1991) A prospective study of indixes predicting the outcome of trials of weaning from mechanical ventilation. NEJM 324: 1445–1450

[13] Macintyre NR, Leatherman NE (1990) Ventilatory muscle loads and the frequency-tidal volume pattern during inspiratory pressure-assisted (pressure-supported) ventilation. Am Rev Respir Dis 141: 327–331

[14] Rotello LC, Warren J, Jastremski MS, Milewski A (1992) A nurse-directed protocol using pulse oximetry to wean mechanically ventilated patients from toxic oxygen concentrations. Chest 102: 1833–1835

[15] Register SD, Downs JB, Stock MC, Kirby RR (1987) Is 50% oxygen harmful? Crit Care Med 15: 598–601

[16] Cane RD, Peruzzi WT, Shapiro BA (1991) Airway pressure release ventilation in the severe acute respiratory failure. Chest 100: 460–463

[17] Tobin MJ (1991) What should the clinician do when a patient "fights the ventilator"? Respiratory Care 36: 395–406

[18] Bersten AD, Rutten AJ, Vedig AE, Skowronski GA (1989) Additional work of breathing imposed by endotracheal tubes, breathing circuits, and intensive care ventilators. Crit Care Med 17

[19] Hoffman RA, Krieger BP, Kramer MR, Segel S, Bizousky F, Gazeroglu H, Sackner MA (1989) End-tidal carbon dioxide in critically ill patients during changes in mechanical ventilation. Am Rev Respir Dis 140: 1265–1268

Knowledge-Based Monitoring and Therapy Planning in Intensive Care Units (ICUs)

S. Miksch[1], W. Horn[1,2], C. Popow[3], and F. Paky[4]

[1] Austrian Research Institute for Artificial Intelligence (ÖFAI),
[2] Department of Medical Cybernetics and Artificial Intelligence,
University of Vienna,
[3] Department of Pediatrics, NICU, University of Vienna,
[4] Gottfried von Preyer Children's Hospital, Vienna, Austria

1. Introduction

This presentation will focus on the special applications of AI technologies in Intensive Care Units (ICUs), and here especially on knowledge-based monitoring and therapy planning systems for artificial ventilator management. Such systems span the range from raw patient signals to sophisticated control decisions, such as filtering out spurious and erroneous data (data validation), real-time operations, and the reactive reconfiguration of the monitoring process as new demands arise (therapy planning).

The care of critically ill patients in ICUs is increasingly complex, involving interpretation of many variables, comparative evaluation of many therapy options, and control of many patient-management parameters. The increasing demand for information storage, retrieval and processing creates problems of information management due to the increased sophistication of laboratory and monitoring equipment. The technical improvement of the ICUs' equipment makes a huge amount of measurements available to the medical staff, and even skilled physicians frequently suffer from these information overload. During the past decade, several knowledge-based systems were introduced to support clinicians with the monitoring of critical care patients and to assist them with diagnostic decisions and therapy planning. These systems range from simple intelligent alarms to sophisticated systems for anesthesia monitoring or ventilator management.

Among other approaches, like statistical analysis, knowledge-based system technology may appropriately represent and organize the practical and theoretical knowledge of experienced specialists and help to cope with information overload with continuous data selection, data validation and therapy planning [15]. But there are known needs and challenges for effective, useful intelligent monitoring and therapy planning systems.

Beginning with the needs of developing knowledge-based monitoring and therapy planning systems. we will give an overview about existing systems in the field of artificial ventilation management systems. Finally, we will summarize the most important challenges for knowledge-based monitoring and control systems.

2. The Need for Knowledge-Based Monitoring and Therapy Planning Systems

Motivations for the development of knowledge-based systems for ICUs are numerous. The most pressing arise from the data overload available from the enormous technological improvements of the technical equipment in ICUs. Even experienced physicians have difficulties facing the important and relevant continuous data and reacting in a time-constraint, critical situation. But these problems are not unique to clinical medicine.

Artificial ventilation has greatly contributed to improve the mortality and morbidity of premature newborn infants [9, 17]. Improved patient monitoring techniques and enhanced knowledge about the pathophysiological mechanisms of barotrauma and oxygen toxicity led to the development of patient-tailored strategies of mechanical ventilation and helped to reduce harmful side effects of respirator therapy. However, the bulk of continuous information arising from complex monitoring systems creates a rising information management problem at Neonatal Intensive Care Units (NICUs).

Not only the amount of information to be processed limits the quality of intensive care, but also human factors, like the problem of vigilance, varying expertise, and human errors. These frequently lead to errors in diagnosis and selection of appropriate treatments.

Knowledge-based system technology may appropriately represent and organize the practical and theoretical knowledge of experienced specialists. Such a system should therefore be able to support the less experienced physician in the complex decision-making of patient care, and the experienced physician in handling and analysing the complex data arising steadily from the patient monitoring system. During the past decade, several knowledge-based systems were introduced. In the next chapter we will give a short overview about intelligent patient monitoring and therapy planning projects in the field of optimizing artificial ventilation.

3. Knowledge-Based Systems for Artificial Ventilation

A pioneer work in the area of knowledge-based monitoring and therapy planning systems was the Ventilator Manager (VM) of Fagan [7]. VM was developed in the late 1970s as one of a series of experiments studying the effectiveness of the MYCIN formalism. VM was designed for an on-line interpretation of quantitative data arising at an ICU in order to manage postsurgical mechanically ventilated patients.

VMS [3] is a ventilator therapy planning system for neonates. Its main features are a complete record keeping facility with log reports and patients' lists and a statistical trend analysis for assisting ventilator adjustment. VMS is based on an implemented algorithm representing conventional therapy for neonates with respiratory distress syndrome and offers additional features such as a graphical display of pressure waveforms and shifted oxygen dissociation curves.

VentPlan [13,14] is a ventilator monitoring and therapy planning system which combines qualitative and quantitative techniques. It is composed of a mathematical modeling section based on equations that describe the physiology of the heart and the lung functions, of a belief network that estimates parameter values by using qualitative information, of a plan evaluator that ranks therapy plans based on a multiattribute scoring system, and of a control algorithm.

COMPAS [16] is a computerized advice giving system designed to assist in the respiratory therapy of patients with adult respiratory syndrome.

Arroe [1] developed a therapy planning system for ventilating neonates. This system proposes the direction of change of the ventilator settings based on actual arterial blood gas samples and ventilator settings. It includes a continuous trend evaluation of the last six blood gas measurements.

SIMON [18, 19] is a ventilator monitoring system for premature infants. It addressed two issues, which up to then had only been covered unsatisfactorily: the issue of context sensitivity, wherein the understanding of the patient's status is related to the pathophysiology of existing disorders, and other internal and external factors such as age or degree of immaturity. The other issue deals with the correctness of measurements.

The Guardian system [10, 11, 2] is a real-time monitoring and therapy planning system which may be applied to respiratory and cardiovascular monitoring problems at surgical ICUs. Guardian simultaneously interprets several channels of real-time data by reactively constructing and modifying its control plans, and interleaving various signal processing tasks according to their relative importance. It is a 'proof of concept' system, which was not designed for practical use.

A small number of systems was designed mainly for intelligent alarming and alarm validating (RESPAID [5], PONI [8]). The major goal of these systems is a reduction in the number of false alarms.

From the practical point of view, the usability of all these systems is limited as concerns their monitoring and therapy planning components. Most systems use invasively determined blood gas measurements for therapy planning, which, however, are only discontinuously and infrequently determined. Moreover, therapy planning in a modern ICU is increasingly based on noninvasive continuous measurements of transcutaneous partial pressure of oxygen ($PtcO_2$), arterial oxygen saturation (SaO_2) and transcutaneous partial pressure of carbon dioxide ($PtcCO_2$). Another problem of the described systems is that they do not allow for individual strategies of artificial ventilation. In addition, data validation modules are simple, and reasoning about the change of parameters over time is missing.

We developed the knowledge-based monitoring and therapy planning system VIE-VENT [12] at the Austrian Research Institute for Artificial Intelligence (ÖFAI) in cooperation with the Gottfried von Preyer Children's Hospital, the Neonatal Intensive Care Unit (NICU) of the Department of Pediatrics of Vienna's University Medical School, and the Department of Medical Cybernetics and Artificial Intelligence, University of Vienna. Developing VIE-VENT, we tried to overcome the limitations of the existing systems. VIE-VENT is specifically designed for practical use under real-time constraints in the NICUs. A context sensitive data validation and therapy planning component were implemented according to practical clinical and textbook knowledge. VIE-VENT uses continuous and discontinuous data input from the patient's monitors, ventilators and the data management systems. VIE-VENT samples transcutaneous measurements and ventilator settings every 10 seconds. The arithmetic means of these 10-second data are stored every 10 minutes for further analysis.

The therapy planning component of VIE-VENT is based on a combination of transcutaneous and invasive blood gas measurements and qualitative clinical observations (e.g. chest wall expansion). The background knowledge for formulating therapy recommendations is a simplified model of neonatal respiration. This model includes the neonates' delay-time of a physiological reaction to an executed therapy action. Therapy recommendations are released depending on various conditions (e. g., depending on the severity of the neonate's ventilatory status, on newly available blood gas analyses, or on various time dependencies). They consist of a set of possible and necessary changes of ventilator settings. The different strategies of these changes are represented according to the degree of blood gas abnormality. We included three possible dynamics of ventilation (e.g. conservative), according to different strategies of therapy planning, in order to be able to fulfill the requirements of different physicians using the system. Another very important feature of VIE-VENT is that in case of a poor condition of the neonate, the dynamics of ventilation is automatically set to aggressive. This represents the practical behavior at a NICU, where the physicians have to react to a deterioration of the patient as quickly and much as possible, in order to rapidly improve the situation. At this time, VIE-VENT is clinically tested at two different NICUs.

4. Some Challenges

The heart of the challenge to medical Artificial Intelligence (AI) applications is the ability to identify and satisfy fundamental clinical needs. There are different ways to cope with this challenge. On the one hand, there is a steady effort concentrating on the technical aspects of diagnosis, monitoring and control of physiological signals. On the other hand, there is a large literature on human factors in the clinical workspace, identifying causes of suboptimal performance and suggesting areas in which such applications might be appropriate [6]. Additionally, there is a large amount of literature on the cognitive aspects of process control [20]. Unfortunately, no really important progress can be achieved with work focusing solely on technical issues. Necessarily, as the technical aspects of the domain start to become clearer, it may now be an appropriate time to undertake a closer examination of the clinical needs that orginally motivated the field of medical AI. This claim gives rise to the problem of cooperation and coordination between medical experts and computer scientists.

Collaboration between physicians and computer scientists is essential for the development of sophisticated knowledge-based systems. Generally, computer scientists have only little clinical experience, and physicians have a poor understanding of computer science. As there are only a few experts with an equal background in medical and computer sciences, both disciplines have to collaborate intensively during the development process, especially during the knowledge acquisition task. Physicians need to structure their "art" of reasoning and decision making. Computer scientists have to accept that "clinical rules" are often based on personal experience, "feelings", sometimes contradictory clinical studies, that very often a third variable which is difficult to assess and to handle, such as the magnitude of the pulmonary perfusion, has a greater influence than all other variables, and that rules and strategies may even change during the developmental process. These difficulties may be overcome only by the fact that both groups are aiming to build a useful application.

For effective therapy planning the validation of data is an essential part, such as handling of noisy and missing data and recognizing artifacts. The recognition of artifacts is a rather complicated task. An artifact is a situation where the measured values do not reflect the clinical context. Several monitors have a built-in module for recognizing artifacts, especially those arising from hardware problems. But the whole data validation cannot be handled by the monitors themselves, and has to be implemented in the monitoring component of the system. There are different methods for detecting artifacts, like the measurement is out of range, which is already covered in the checking the plausibility of measurements, rapid oscillations or very fast changing of a single measurement, cross relations between different measurements.

Much work has been focused on supporting clinicians with diagnosis, and less on the control or therapy planning task. This is surprising, since much of the patient care activity in ICUs is associated with control. Therefore systems which assist clinicians in making an assessment of monitored data may be more useful than systems that attempt to manufacture diagnosis. In other words, it may well be the case that the majority of physicians do not have difficulty in making a diagnosis, but rather in establishing a clear picture of the state of the world, and clarifying their goals and assumptions, prior to attempting to make a diagnosis. If this is really the case, then assessment is the key bottleneck. This should influence the design of supporting systems for monitoring and therapy planning.

While much work goes into the design of the computational components of monitoring and therapy planning, little is thought about the visualization of relevant clinical data, the importance of the design of a user-friendly and functional user-interface. It should be a priority for systems designers to explicitly identify the clinician tasks, the relevant functionality of the needed interface, and the manner in which clinicians will successfully use such a system. Otherwise the acceptance of the system would be very low.

To increase the acceptance of such a system there are a lot of other claims, like the model behind the system should be as clear as possible for the user of the system. We should avoid the introduction of excessive complexity, or oversimplification in the conceptual model. On the other hand knowledge-based systems should be practically oriented. The various module components should be built in analogy to the clinical reasoning process. There should be enough time to train the medical staff in using the system and in understanding the reasoning process of the system. Finally, another great issue is the minimization of the user's input and the integration of the monitoring and therapy planning system in the frequently existing patient data management system.

Finally, we should not forget how important and essential the technical, empirical and subjective evaluation of such knowledge-based systems is. Coping with problems, like finding independent experts who are willing to join the evaluation task, testing logical consistency, logical and functional completeness, reliability, robustness, accuracy and adequacy of the knowledge base, proving security and performance of the system.

Our underlying motivation for developing knowledge-based monitoring and therapy planning systems should be to improve the clinical

S. Miksch et al.

outcome. The clearer our understanding of the place of intelligent monitoring and therapy planning system in the clinical workspace is, the more effective and functional will be our systems.

Acknowledgement

The project VIE-VENT is supported by the "Medizinisch-Wissenschaftlicher Fonds" of the Mayor of the City of Vienna, Austria. We also greatly appreciate the support given to the Austrian Research Institute for Artificial Intelligence (ÖFAI) by the Austrian Federal Ministry of Science and Research, Vienna.

References

[1] Arroe M (1991) A computerized aid in ventilating neonates. Computers Biol Med 21: 15–21
[2] Ash D, Gold G, Seiver A, Hayes-Roth B (1993) Guaranteeing real-time response with limited resources. Artificial Intelligence in Medicine 5: 49–66
[3] Boyarsky A (1987) Computerized ventilation management system for neonates. Journal of Perinatology 7: 21–29
[4] Coiera E (1993) Intelligent monitoring and control of physiological systems, editorial. Artificial Intelligence in Medicine 5: 1–8
[5] Chambrin MC, Chopin C, Ravaux P, Mangalaboyi J, Lestavel P, Fourrier F (1989) RESPAID: Computer-aided decision support for respiratory data in ICU. Proc. Eleventh Annual Conf. IEEE Engineering in Medicine and Biology Soc., Seattle, WA.
[6] Fafchamps D, Young C, Tang P (1991) Modelling work practices: Input to the design of physician's workstation. In: Proceedings of 15th Symposium on Computer Applications in Medical Care, Washington, DC, pp 788–792
[7] Fagan LM, Shortliffe EH, Buchanan BG (1980) Computer-based medical decision making: From MYCIN to VM. Automedica 3: 97–106
[8] Grafinkel D, Matsiras PV, Lecky JH, Aukburg SJ, Matschinsky BB, Mavrides TG (1988) PONI: An intelligent alarm system for respiratory and circulation management in the operating room. Proc. 12th Annual Symp. Comput. Appl. Med. Care, Washington, DC
[9] Goldsmith JP, Karotkin EH (1988) Assisted ventilation of the neonates. Saunders, Philadelphia
[10] Hayes-Roth B, Washington R, Hewett M, Seiver A (1989) Intelligent monitoring and control. In: Proceedings of the Eleventh International Joint Conference on Artificial Intelligence (IJCAI-89). Morgan Kaufmann, Los Altos, CA, pp 243–249
[11] Hayes-Roth B, Washington R, Ash D, Hewett M, Collinot A, Vina A, Seiver A (1992) Guardian: A prototype intelligent agent for intensive-care monitoring. Artificial Intelligence in Medicine 4: 165–185

[12] Miksch S, Horn W, Popow C, Paky F (1993) VIE-VENT: Knowledge-based monitoring and therapy planning of the artificial ventilation of newborn infants. In: Proc. AIME-93, Munich, Germany

[13] Rutledge G, Thomsen G, Beinlich I, Farr B, Sheiner L, Fagan LM (1989) Combining qualitative and quantitative computation in a ventilator therapy planner. Proc. 13th Annual Symp. Comput. Appl. Med. Care, Washington, DC

[14] Rutledge GW, Thomsen GE, Farr BR, Tovar MA, Polaschek JX, Beinlich IA, Sheiner LB, Fagan LM (1993) The design and implementation of a ventilator-management advisor. Artificial Intelligence in Medicine 5: 67–82

[15] Shortliffe EH (1991) Knowledge-based system in medicine. In: Proc. Medical Informatics Europe 1991. Springer, Berlin

[16] Sitting DF, Pace NL, Gardner RM, Morris AH, Wallace J (1990) Clinical evaluation of computer-based respiratory care algorithms. Int. Journal of Clinical Monitoring and Computing 7: 177–185

[17] Teberg AJ, Hodgman JE (1992) Survival of infants with birthweight 500–1500 g. In: Lucey JF (ed) Hot topics in neonatology. Proc. Ross Lab. Special Conference

[18] Uckun S, Dawant BM (1992) Qualitative modelling as a paradigm for diagnosis and prediction in critical care environments. Artificial Intelligence in Medicine 4: 127–144

[19] Uckun S, Dawant BM, Lindstrom DP (1993) Model-based diagnosis in intensive care monitoring: The YAQ approach. Artificial Intelligence in Medicine 5: 31–48

[20] Wickens CD (1992) Engineering psychology and human performance. Harper Collins, New York

Authors

Doz. Dr. K. P. Adlassnig, University of Vienna, Institute for Medical Computer Sciences, Währinger Gürtel 18–20, A-1090 Vienna, Austria

Dr. H. Andel, University of Vienna, Department of Anaesthesia and General Intensive Care, Währinger Gürtel 18–20, A-1090 Vienna, Austria

Dr. E. Donner, University of Vienna, Department of Cardiothoracic Anaesthesia and Intensive Care Medicine, Währinger Gürtel 18–20, A-1090 Vienna, Austria

Dipl.-Ing. J. Gamper, University of Vienna, Institute for Medical Computer Sciences, Währinger Gürtel 18–20, A-1090 Vienna, Austria

Prof. Dr. W. Haider, University of Vienna, Department of Cardiothoracic Anaesthesia and Intensive Care Medicine, Währinger Gürtel 18–20, A-1090 Vienna, Austria

A. Heikelä, MD, Clinisoft LTD, Teknia Science Park, Savilahdentie 6, FIN-70211 Kuopio, Finland

Dr. D. Heilinger, University of Vienna, Department of Cardiothoracic Anaesthesia and Intensive Care Medicine, Währinger Gürtel 18–20, A-1090 Vienna, Austria

Dr. M. Hiesmayr, University of Vienna, Department of Cardiothoracic Anaesthesia and Intensive Care Medicine, Währinger Gürtel 18–20, A-1090 Vienna, Austria

Dipl.-Ing. J. Hiller, Clinic for Anaesthesiology, Intensive Care Medicine and Pain Therapy, Klinik am Eichert, Postfach 660, D-73006 Göppingen, Germany

Doz. Dr. W. Horn, University of Vienna, Department of Medical Cybernetics and Artificial Intelligence, Austrian Research Institute for Artificial Intelligence (ÖFAI), Schottengasse 3, A-1010 Vienna, Austria

Dr. M. Imhoff, Chirurgische Klinik, Städtische Kliniken, Dortmund, Germany

Dr. P. Keznickl, University of Vienna, Department of Cardiothoracic Anaesthesia and Intensive Care Medicine, Währinger Gürtel 18–20, A-1090 Vienna, Austria

Prof. Dr. K. Lenz, University of Vienna, Department of Inner Medicine IV, ICU 13H1, Währinger Gürtel 18–20, A-1090 Vienna, Austria

Dr. P. Mares, University of Vienna, Department of Cardiothoracic Anaesthesia and Intensive Care Medicine, Währinger Gürtel 18–20, A-1090 Vienna, Austria

Dr. J. Martin, Clinic for Anaesthesiology, Intensive Care Medicine and Pain Therapy, Klinik am Eichert, Postfach 660, D-73006 Göppingen, Germany

Dr. M. Messelken, Clinic for Anaesthesiology, Intensive Care Medicine and Pain Therapy, Klinik am Eichert, Postfach 660, D-73006 Göppingen, Germany

DDr. P. G. H. Metnitz, University of Vienna, Department of Inner Medicine IV, ICU 13H1, Währinger Gürtel 18–20, A-1090 Vienna, Austria

Dr. S. Miksch, Austrian Research Institute for Artificial Intelligence (ÖFAI), Schottengasse 3, A-1010 Vienna, Austria

Prof. Dr. P. Milewski, Clinic for Anaesthesiology, Intensive Care Medicine and Pain Therapy, Klinik am Eichert, Postfach 660, D-73006 Göppingen, Germany

Dr. T. Neugebauer, University of Vienna, Department of Cardiothoracic Anaesthesia and Intensive Care Medicine, Research Institute for Intensive Care Medicine, Währinger Gürtel 18–20, A-1090 Vienna, Austria

A. Nyberg, Clinisoft LTD, Teknia Science Park, Savilahdentie 6, FIN-70211 Kuopio, Finland

Dr. F. Paky, Gottfried v. Preyer's Children's Hospital, Schankenberggasse 31, A-1110 Vienna, Austria

Ing. W. Perkmann, Hewlett Packard Medical Systems Group, Lieblgasse 1, A-1220 Vienna, Austria

Doz. Dr. C. Popow, University of Vienna, Department of Pediatrics, NICU, Währinger Gürtel 18–20, A-1090 Vienna, Austria

Dr. G. Schak, Hewlett Packard Medical Systems Group, Lieblgasse 1, A-1220 Vienna, Austria

Dr. H. Vedovelli, Hewlett Packard Medical Systems Group, Lieblgasse 1, A-1220 Vienna, Austria

DKS J. Wilding, University of Vienna, Department of Inner Medicine IV, ICU 13H1, Währinger Gürtel 18–20, A-1090 Vienna, Austria

Dr. P. Zwölfer, University of Vienna, Department of Cardiothoracic Anaesthesia and Intensive Care Medicine, Währinger Gürtel 18–20, A-1090 Vienna, Austria

Clinisoft LTD, Teknia Science Park, Savilahdentie 6, FIN-70211 Kuopio, Finland

Hewlett Packard Medical Systems Group, Lieblgasse 1, A-1220 Vienna, Austria

Siemens AG, Bereich Medizinische Technik, Henkestrasse 127, D-91052 Erlangen, Germany

Erwin Deutsch, Gunther Kleinberger, Kurt Lenz,
Rudolf Ritz, Bruno Schneeweiß, Hans-Peter Schuster,
Georg Simbruner, Jörg Slany (Hrsg.)

Multiorganversagen

10. Wiener Intensivmedizinische Tage, 21.-22. Februar 1992

1992. 20 Abbildungen. VII, 184 Seiten.
Broschiert öS 420,–, DM 59,–. 3-211-82334-4
(Intensivmedizinisches Seminar, Band 4)

Preisänderungen vorbehalten

Das Multiorganversagen stellt eine der größten Herausforderungen in der Intensivmedizin dar. Aufgrund ausgedehnter Forschungstätigkeit konnten in den letzten Jahren neue Erkenntnisse in der Entstehung dieses bedrohlichen Krankheitsbildes und in dessen Beherrschung gewonnen werden. Hauptthema der 10. Wiener Intensivmedizinischen Tage war daher das Multiorganversagen, dessen wichtigste Referate im vorliegenden vierten Band des Intensivmedizinischen Seminars präsentiert werden. Im ersten Teil wird auf mögliche Ursachen wie Sepsis und Polytrauma eingegangen, wobei in einem eigenen Kapitel das Versagen der Zelle im Rahmen dieses Krankheitsbildes dargestellt wird. Der zweite Teil behandelt das Versagen der einzelnen Organe im Rahmen des Multiorganversagens. Im dritten Teil werden die Überwachungsmöglichkeiten von Organfunktionen und deren klinische Relevanz diskutiert, und schließlich wird im letzten Teil des Buches auf die Therapie des Patienten im Multiorganversagen eingegangen.

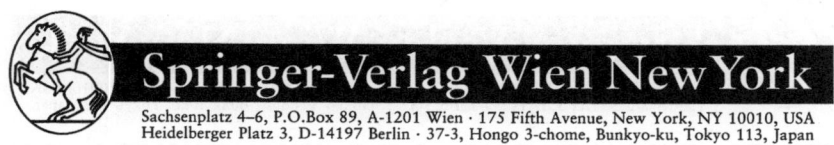
Springer-Verlag Wien New York

Sachsenplatz 4–6, P.O.Box 89, A-1201 Wien · 175 Fifth Avenue, New York, NY 10010, USA
Heidelberger Platz 3, D-14197 Berlin · 37-3, Hongo 3-chome, Bunkyo-ku, Tokyo 113, Japan

Gunther Kleinberger, Kurt Lenz, Rudolf Ritz,
Hans-Peter Schuster, Georg Simbruner, Jörg Slany (Hrsg.)

Beatmung

1993. 16 Abbildungen. VII, 145 Seiten.
Broschiert öS 345,–, DM 49,–. ISBN 3-211-82438-3
(Intensivmedizinisches Seminar, Band 5)

Preisänderungen vorbehalten

Die respiratorische Insuffizienz stellt eines der zentralen
Probleme des Patienten auf der Intensivstation dar. Durch
Verbesserung der Technik in der maschinellen Beatmung
und in den augmentierenden Verfahren sowie in der
medikamentösen Therapie ist es in den letzten Jahren
gelungen, große Fortschritte in der Behandlung dieser
Patienten zu erzielen. In diesem Band sind die wichtigsten
Vorträge der 11. Wiener Intensivmedizinischen Tage, deren
Hauptthema die Beatmung war, dargestellt. Neben der
Pathophysiologie der Beatmung wird die Therapie bei den
verschiedenen Ursachen der respiratorischen Insuffizienz
abgehandelt. Es werden hierbei die verschiedenen Formen
der Beatmung und die medikamentösen Therapien, wie die
Applikation des Surfactant beim Frühgeborenen und beim
Erwachsenen sowie die NO Therapie beim Patienten mit
ARDS dargestellt. Weiters werden das Für und Wider der
Hämofiltration als unterstützende Therapie und die extra-
korporale CO_2 Elimination diskutiert. Insgesamt soll dieses
Buch den aktuellen Stand der wichtigsten Therapiemöglich-
keiten bei der respiratorischen Insuffizienz sowie praktisch
relevante Information für den Intensivmediziner bieten.

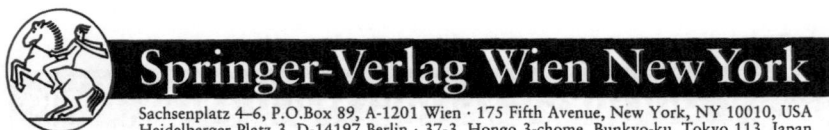
Springer-Verlag Wien New York

Sachsenplatz 4–6, P.O.Box 89, A-1201 Wien · 175 Fifth Avenue, New York, NY 10010, USA
Heidelberger Platz 3, D-14197 Berlin · 37-3, Hongo 3-chome, Bunkyo-ku, Tokyo 113, Japan